Adolescent Sexuality

Editor

MARIANNE E. FELICE

PEDIATRIC CLINICS
OF NORTH AMERICA

www.pediatric.theclinics.com

Consulting Editor
BONITA F. STANTON

April 2017 • Volume 64 • Number 2

ELSEVIER

1600 John F. Kennedy Boulevard • Suite 1800 • Philadelphia, Pennsylvania, 19103-2899

http://www.theclinics.com

THE PEDIATRIC CLINICS OF NORTH AMERICA Volume 64, Number 2
April 2017 ISSN 0031-3955, ISBN-13: 978-0-323-52421-6

Editor: Kerry Holland
Developmental Editor: Casey Potter

The Pediatric Clinics of North America (ISSN 0031-3955) is published bimonthly by Elsevier Inc., 360 Park Avenue South, New York, NY 10010-1710. Months of issue are February, April, June, August, October, and December. Periodicals postage paid at New York, NY and additional mailing offices. Subscription prices are $208.00 per year (US individuals), $589.00 per year (US institutions), $281.00 per year (Canadian individuals), $784.00 per year (Canadian institutions), $338.00 per year (international individuals), $784.00 per year (international institutions), $100.00 per year (US students and residents), and $165.00 per year (international and Canadian residents and students). To receive students/resident rare, orders must be accompanied by name of affiliated institution, date of term, and the signature of program/residency coordinator on institution letterhead. Orders will be billed at individual rate until proof of status is received. Foreign air speed delivery is included in all *Clinics* subscription prices. All prices are subject to change without notice. **POSTMASTER:** Send address changes to *The Pediatric Clinics of North America*, Elsevier Health Sciences Division, Subscription Customer Service, 3251 Riverport Lane, Maryland Heights, MO 63043. **Customer Service: 1-800-654-2452 (US and Canada). From outside of the US and Canada: 1-314-447-8871. Fax: 1-314-447-8029. For print support, E-mail: JournalsCustomerService-usa@elsevier.com. For online support, E-mail: JournalsOnlineSupport-usa@elsevier.com**.

Reprints. For copies of 100 or more, of articles in this publication, please contact the Commercial Reprints Department, Elsevier Inc., 360 Park Avenue South, New York, NY 10010-1710. Tel.: 212-633-3874; Fax: 212-633-3820; E-mail: reprints@elsevier.com.

The Pediatric Clinics of North America is also published in Spanish by McGraw-Hill Inter-americana Editores S.A., Mexico City, Mexico; in Portuguese by Riechmann and Affonso Editores, Rua Comandante Coelho 1085, CEP 21250, Rio de Janeiro, Brazil; and in Greek by Althayia SA, Athens, Greece.

The Pediatric Clinics of North America is covered in *MEDLINE/PubMed (Index Medicus), Excerpta Medica, Current Contents, Current Contents/Clinical Medicine, Science Citation Index, ASCA, ISI/BIOMED,* and *BIOSIS.*

PROGRAM OBJECTIVE
The goal of the *Pediatric Clinics of North America* is to keep practicing physicians and residents up to date with current clinical practice in pediatrics by providing timely articles reviewing the state-of-the-art in patient care.

TARGET AUDIENCE
All practicing pediatricians, physicians and healthcare professionals who provide patient care to pediatric patients.

LEARNING OBJECTIVES
Upon completion of this activity, participants will be able to:
1. Review updates in concepts in adolescent sexuality.
2. Discuss pregnancy and contraception methods in adolescents.
3. Recognize issues in adolescent sexuality such as sex trafficking, sexual violence, and treating youth in the juvenile justice system.

ACCREDITATION
The Elsevier Office of Continuing Medical Education (EOCME) is accredited by the Accreditation Council for Continuing Medical Education (ACCME) to provide continuing medical education for physicians.

The EOCME designates this enduring material for a maximum of 15 *AMA PRA Category 1 Credit*(s)™. Physicians should claim only the credit commensurate with the extent of their participation in the activity.

All other health care professionals requesting continuing education credit for this enduring material will be issued a certificate of participation.

DISCLOSURE OF CONFLICTS OF INTEREST
The EOCME assesses conflict of interest with its instructors, faculty, planners, and other individuals who are in a position to control the content of CME activities. All relevant conflicts of interest that are identified are thoroughly vetted by EOCME for fair balance, scientific objectivity, and patient care recommendations. EOCME is committed to providing its learners with CME activities that promote improvements or quality in healthcare and not a specific proprietary business or a commercial interest.

The planning committee, staff, authors and editors listed below have identified no financial relationships or relationships to products or devices they or their spouse/life partner have with commercial interest related to the content of this CME activity:
Suzanne Allen, MSN, RN, CPNP-PC; Marcus Vinicius Ortega Alves, MD; Amie M. Ashcraft, PHD, MPH; Erin Barlow, MD; Christine E. Barron, MD; Gale R. Burnstein, MD, MPH; Taylor Rose Ellsworth, MPH; Marianne E. Felice, MD; Anjali Fortna; Kerry Holland; Cynthia Holland-Hall, MD, MPH; Vanessa Issac, MD; Dana Kaplan, MD; Indu Kumari; Heidi K. Leftwich, DO; Elizabeth Miller, MD, PhD; Jessica L. Moore, BA; Pamela J. Murray, MD, MHP; Betsy Pfeffer, MD; Anne Powell, MD; Elisabeth H. Quint, MD; Sheryl A. Ryan, MD; Ann L. Sattler, MD, MAT; Bonita F. Stanton, MD; Zoon Wangu, MD; Katie Widmeier; Amy Williams.

The planning committee, staff, authors and editors listed below have identified financial relationships or relationships to products or devices they or their spouse/life partner have with commercial interest related to the content of this CME activity:
Diane R. Blake, MD receives royalties/patents from UpToDate, Ino.
Melanie A. Gold, DO, DMQ is a consultant/advisor for Bayer AG and Afaxys, Inc, and receives royalties/patents from Oxford University Press.
Amy M. Middleman, MD, MSEd, MPH receives royalties/patents from UpToDate, Inc.
Ellen S. Rome, MD, MPH is on the speakers' bureau for, and is a consultant/advisor for, Merck & Co., Inc.

UNAPPROVED/OFF-LABEL USE DISCLOSURE
The EOCME requires CME faculty to disclose to the participants:
1. When products or procedures being discussed are off-label, unlabelled, experimental, and/or investigational (not US Food and Drug Administration [FDA] approved); and
2. Any limitations on the information presented, such as data that are preliminary or that represent ongoing research, interim analyses, and/or unsupported opinions. Faculty may discuss information about pharmaceutical agents that is outside of FDA-approved labelling. This information is intended solely for CME

and is not intended to promote off-label use of these medications. If you have any questions, contact the medical affairs department of the manufacturer for the most recent prescribing information.

TO ENROLL
To enroll in the *Pediatric Clinics of North America* Continuing Medical Education program, call customer service at 1-800-654-2452 or sign up online at http://www.theclinics.com/home/cme. The CME program is available to subscribers for an additional annual fee of USD 290.

METHOD OF PARTICIPATION
In order to claim credit, participants must complete the following:
1. Complete enrolment as indicated above.
2. Read the activity.
3. Complete the CME Test and Evaluation. Participants must achieve a score of 70% on the test. All CME Tests and Evaluations must be completed online.

CME INQUIRIES/SPECIAL NEEDS
For all CME inquiries or special needs, please contact elsevierCME@elsevier.com.

Contributors

CONSULTING EDITOR

BONITA F. STANTON, MD
Founding Dean, School of Medicine, Professor of Pediatrics, Seton Hall University, South Orange, New Jersey

EDITOR

MARIANNE E. FELICE, MD
Professor of Pediatrics and Obstetrics/Gynecology, University of Massachusetts Medical School, Worcester, Massachusetts

AUTHORS

SUZANNE ALLEN, MSN, RN, CPNP-PC
Division of Adolescent Medicine, Department of Pediatrics, UMass Memorial Children's Medical Center, Worcester, Massachusetts

MARCUS VINICIUS ORTEGA ALVES, MD
Department of Obstetrics and Gynecology, University of Massachusetts Medical School, Worcester, Massachusetts

AMIE M. ASHCRAFT, PhD, MPH
Research Manager, Department of Pediatrics, West Virginia University School of Medicine, Morgantown, West Virginia

ERIN BARLOW, MD
Division of Adolescent Gynecology, Department of Obstetrics/Gynecology; Division of Adolescent Medicine, Department of Pediatrics, University of Massachusetts Medical School, Worcester, Massachusetts

CHRISTINE E. BARRON, MD
Aubin Child Protection Center, Hasbro Children's Hospital; Department of Pediatrics, The Warren Alpert Medical School of Brown University, Providence, Rhode Island

DIANE R. BLAKE, MD
Professor, Department of Pediatrics, University of Massachusetts Medical School, Worcester, Massachusetts

GALE R. BURSTEIN, MD, MPH
Clinical Professor of Pediatrics, Division of Adolescent Medicine, SUNY at Buffalo School of Medicine and Biomedical Sciences, Erie County Department of Health, Buffalo, New York; New York City STD/HIV Prevention Training Center, New York, New York

TAYLOR ROSE ELLSWORTH, MPH
Director, Education, Research and Training, Physicians for Reproductive Health, New York, New York

MELANIE A. GOLD, DO, DMQ
Professor of Pediatrics and Professor of Population and Family Health, Center for Community and Health Education, Columbia University Medical Center, New York, New York

CYNTHIA HOLLAND-HALL, MD, MPH
Associate Professor of Pediatrics, Section of Adolescent Medicine, Nationwide Children's Hospital, The Ohio State University College of Medicine, Columbus, Ohio

VERONICA ISSAC, MD
Staff Physician, Center for Adolescent Medicine, Cleveland Clinic Children's Hospital, Cleveland, Ohio

DANA M. KAPLAN, MD
Division of Child Abuse and Neglect, Department of Pediatrics, Staten Island University Hospital, Staten Island, New York

HEIDI K. LEFTWICH, DO
Division of Maternal-Fetal Medicine, Department of Obstetrics and Gynecology, University of Massachusetts Medical School, Worcester, Massachusetts

AMY B. MIDDLEMAN, MD, MSEd, MPH
Professor, Department of Pediatrics, University of Oklahoma Health Sciences Center, Oklahoma City, Oklahoma

ELIZABETH MILLER, MD, PhD
Division of Adolescent and Young Adult Medicine, Professor of Pediatrics, Children's Hospital of Pittsburgh of UPMC, University of Pittsburgh School of Medicine, Pittsburgh, Pennsylvania

JESSICA L. MOORE, BA
Aubin Child Protection Center, Hasbro Children's Hospital, Providence, Rhode Island

PAMELA J. MURRAY, MD, MHP
Professor, Department of Pediatrics, West Virginia University School of Medicine, Morgantown, West Virginia

BETSY PFEFFER, MD
Associate Professor of Pediatrics at Columbia University Medical Center, Division of Child & Adolescent Health, New York, New York

ANNE POWELL, MD
Assistant Professor of Pediatrics, Division of Adolescent Medicine, University of Massachusetts Medical School, Worcester, Massachusetts

ELISABETH H. QUINT, MD
Professor, Obstetrics and Gynecology, University of Michigan Medical School, Ann Arbor, Michigan

ELLEN S. ROME, MD, MPH
Head, Center for Adolescent Medicine, Cleveland Clinic Children's Hospital; Professor of Pediatrics, Cleveland Clinic Lerner College of Medicine, Cleveland, Ohio

SHERYL A. RYAN, MD
Professor of Pediatrics, Section of Adolescent Medicine, Department of Pediatrics, Yale University School of Medicine, New Haven, Connecticut

ANN L. SATTLER, MD, MAT
Clinical Professor of Pediatrics, Division of Adolescent Medicine, University of Massachusetts Medical School, Worcester, Massachusetts

ZOON WANGU, MD
Assistant Professor of Pediatrics, UMass Medical School and Division of Pediatric Infectious Diseases & Immunology, UMass Memorial Children's Medical Center, Worcester, Massachusetts; Clinical Faculty, Ratelle STD/HIV Prevention Training Center, Massachusetts Department of Public Health, Jamaica Plain, Massachusetts

Contents

 Video content accompanies this article at http://www.pediatric.
theclinics.com.

> To optimally address sex and sexuality, normalize gender and sexual di-
> versities, and attend to adolescents' needs, clinicians will best serve their
> patients and their families by becoming comfortable initiating confidential,
> developmentally appropriate discussions with all adolescent patients. The
> goal is to create a safe, affirming, nonjudgmental space wherein adoles-
> cents may learn about sexual matters, discuss concerns, ask questions,
> and find support to assist them to achieve healthy, positive development.
> This article provides useful, practical suggestions to begin these conversa-
> tions, offers specific examples and tips to encourage dialogue, and dis-
> cusses ways to be a resource to adolescent patients.

> This article is intended as a resource for pediatric providers to help them
> guide parents in increasing the quantity and quality of their communication
> about sexuality. The article provides an overview of the best practices asso-
> ciated with parent-adolescent communication about major topics related to
> sexuality (eg, masturbation, contraception, romantic relationships). In addi-
> tionally, the article includes concrete suggestions for parents to improve
> their communication with teens as well as resources for further guidance.

> Rates of cancers attributable to human papillomavirus (HPV) are rising. A
> safe and extremely effective vaccine is available to prevent many of these
> cancers. Studies have shown that health care providers' recommendation
> to immunize is the most important factor in parents' decision. Parents of all
> adolescent boys and girls should receive a strong and unequivocal recom-
> mendation to vaccinate their child against HPV at the 11- or 12-year-old
> well child visit. Ideally, adolescents complete their HPV vaccine series
> by their 13th birthday, leading to greater immune response and protection
> before most adolescents are exposed to sexually transmitted HPV.

seeking a second chance to prevent the unintended consequences of unplanned sexual activity. At present, 5 postcoital methods remain available as EC globally: intrauterine devices, ulipristal acetate, a selective progesterone modulator, mifepristone; levonorgestrel, and ethinyl estradiol plus levonorgestrel or norgestrel (rarely used now that progestin only methods are more readily available).

and brief anticipatory guidance with all adolescent patients about healthy and unhealthy relationships and sexual consent, health care providers can help promote healthy adolescent sexual relationships, ensure youth know about available resources and supports for relationship abuse and sexual violence (including how to help a friend), and facilitate connections to victim service advocates, both for prevention and intervention.

Healthy sexual development is important for adolescents with and without disabilities, yet the topic of sexuality is often ignored in the disabled population. Adolescents with mild or moderate degrees of disability have rates of sexual activity and reproductive health needs comparable to their typically developing peers. Their need for support, risk reduction, and education in sexual health may exceed that of their peers. The medical provider may support healthy sexual development through education, anticipatory guidance, menstrual and contraceptive management, and by expanding the notion of sexuality to include a broader conceptualization of sexual behavior and expression.

Adolescents involved with the juvenile justice system have higher rates of risky sexual behaviors, resulting in high rates of sexually transmitted infections and increased risk of human immunodeficiency virus, early or complicated pregnancy, and parenting issues. Comorbid substance abuse, gang association, mental health issues, and history of having been abused as children result in further elevated rates. Girls and lesbian, gay, bisexual, and transgender youths represent growing subpopulations with special risks. Increasingly diverted to community-based alternatives, juvenile justice–involved teens obtain most of their medical care from community providers, who need to understand their risks to provide appropriate, optimal care.

PEDIATRIC CLINICS OF NORTH AMERICA

THE CLINICS ARE AVAILABLE ONLINE!
Access your subscription at:
www.theclinics.com

Foreword

Adolescents Too Are Not Just "Little Adults"

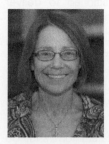

Bonita F. Stanton, MD
Consulting Editor

The field of adolescent medicine has undergone dramatic change over the course of the last several decades, arguably more so than most of the other developmental periods within the purview of the pediatrician. In part, this greater magnitude of change results from the adolescent's exponentially increasing direct interaction with the environment compared with that of younger categories of the "pediatric" subpopulations (preteens, school-aged children, preschool children, toddlers, infants, and neonates).

The adolescent's potential to engage with the environment has been greatly expanded through technology, the social media, globalization, and travel opportunities for junior and senior high school students outside of the purview of their parents. Today's teenager has vastly expanded access to new ideas, new knowledge, and new opportunities, both beneficial and potentially harmful, from across the nation and the globe. The medical community and lay press have emphasized the need for parents to be aware of these pressures, opportunities, and risks, and to develop effective means of communicating with their adolescent children about them. This issue addresses the need not only for *parents* but also for all *pediatricians* to be familiar with the technologies, the social venues, the biologic opportunities, and the hazards open to youth and age-appropriate chaperoning in the twenty-first century. Likewise, significant advances in approaching and talking with adolescents and with minimizing or eliminating the adverse consequences of some of these encounters have been made over the past decades. Again, these advances in our approaches are not just for parents and classroom teachers but also for pediatricians. Fortunately, not only have the causes of diseases impacting adolescents changed and but so too have opportunities to optimize prevention and treatment and to mitigate the short-term and long-term consequences of negative exposures. Finally, in the last two decades, much greater attention has been focused on the criminal practice of human trafficking—even though this activity has existed for decades or longer across the world. Particularly alarming in this regard is the sexual trafficking of teenaged children,

Pediatr Clin N Am 64 (2017) xv–xvi
http://dx.doi.org/10.1016/j.pcl.2017.01.002
0031-3955/17/© 2017 Published by Elsevier Inc.

whether they are adolescents from other countries brought to the United States, US adolescents being trafficked within America, or US teens being trafficked to other countries. Pediatricians must be aware of this abhorrent phenomenon as they may have an opportunity to recognize and intervene on the behalf of these young victims.

All pediatricians must be aware of the range of these potential exposures, diseases, therapies, and communication approaches. After reading this issue and practicing its take-away messages, today's pediatricians will be better positioned to deliver contemporary guidance and care to today's older pediatric patients.

Bonita F. Stanton, MD
School of Medicine
Seton Hall University
400 South Orange Avenue
South Orange, NJ 07079, USA

E-mail address:
bonita.stanton@shu.edu

Preface
A Primer for Primary Care Clinicians Caring for Sexually Active Adolescents

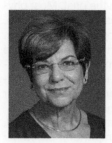

Marianne E. Felice, MD
Editor

This slim issue of thirteen articles was specifically designed with the needs of the General Pediatrician in mind. The list of topics covers a broad scope of clinical issues that are common among adolescent patients, particularly adolescents who are sexually active. Many pediatricians feel poorly equipped to address sexual matters in teens either because they do not have updated knowledge about them or because the issues are complicated and take more time than usually scheduled in a busy practice. This issue will help pediatricians feel more confident caring for their adolescent patients. All the authors have made a concerted effort to provide a concise review of the topic assigned to them coupled with practical suggestions for the clinician to consider.

The first two articles address ways to talk about sex with adolescents and suggestions for talking to parents about their teenager's sexuality. The next article addresses the HPV vaccine and urges primary care clinicians to immunize their young patients. The following article is an excellent review of dysmenorrhea, a very common presenting complaint by teenage girls. The next three articles walk the physician through contraception options for sexually active teens from how to choose the best oral contraceptive pill for a specific teen to recommendations for long-acting reversible contraception (LARC) methods to the use of emergency contraception when needed. It is important to note that both the American Academy of Pediatrics and the American College of Obstetricians/Gynecologists now recommend LARC methods as the first line of contraception for adolescents for whom there are no contraindications. In the next article, the author recommends ways that a general pediatrician can be helpful when one of his/her patients becomes pregnant. Another article in this issue is an excellent summary of the new guidelines for identifying and treating sexually transmitted infections.

Pediatr Clin N Am 64 (2017) xvii–xviii
http://dx.doi.org/10.1016/j.pcl.2017.01.001
0031-3955/17/© 2017 Published by Elsevier Inc.

pediatric.theclinics.com

The last four articles bring attention to special issues that are becoming more important in today's society. Clinicians may not be aware of the disturbing problem of domestic sexual trafficking of minors in the United States. One article urges physicians to be alert for this form of abuse in their practices. Sexual abuse and rape are not uncommon in the adolescent/young adult population, but most of those patients present to emergency rooms for services, not to their physician's office. An article that addresses ways to help young people avoid being a victim of partner violence may be more practical for primary care physicians than an article on rape kits. We now have more young people with disabilities than we have ever had in the past. Most physicians have never been trained in how to address sexual issues in this population. However, in this issue, an article provides a thorough, practical approach to the topic. Last, relatively few pediatricians are involved with adolescents in the juvenile justice system, yet these young people are being returned to their communities from detention facilities on a regular basis, and they have clinical problems related to sexual issues as often if not more than young people who have never been detained. Another article in this issue will help clinicians be more sensitive to their needs as well.

In this issue, we do not address the specific issues related to gay, lesbian, bisexual, or transgender youth. This is not because those issues are not important, but rather because they are so important that a past issue of *Pediatric Clinics of North America* was devoted to that topic alone (Stewart L. Adelson, Nadia L. Dowshen, Harvey J. Makadon, et al. Lesbian, gay, bisexual, and transgender youth. *Pediatr Clin North Am* 2016;63(6)).

Finally, I want to thank all the authors who contributed to this issue for their hard work, enthusiasm, attention to detail, and practical advice they offered the reader in the discussion of their topics. And I want to thank all the clinicians who continue to care for adolescent patients despite the challenges they may give us. Caring for young people is one way that we will all stay young.

Marianne E. Felice, MD
University of Massachusetts Medical School
Department of Pediatrics
55 Lake Avenue North
Worcester, MA 01655, USA

E-mail address:
marianne.felice@umassmemorial.org

Interviewing Adolescents About Sexual Matters

Betsy Pfeffer, MD[a],*, Taylor Rose Ellsworth, MPH[b], Melanie A. Gold, DO, DMQ[c,d]

KEYWORDS

- Adolescent sexuality • Confidentiality • Gender identity • Sexual orientation
- Sexual attraction • Healthy relationships • Sexual behavior

KEY POINTS

- Sexuality is an integral part of adolescent health and development that should be assessed routinely with all adolescents as part of their bio-psychosocial health.
- Interviewing about sexual matters should go beyond inquiring about engaging in sexual behaviors to include gender identity/expression, sexual attraction, sexual orientation identity, and healthy relationships.
- Adolescents need to be interviewed about sexual matters in a developmentally appropriate manner and with confidentiality pre-established.

 Video content accompanies this article at http://www.pediatric.theclinics.com.

INTRODUCTION

Why talk to adolescents about sexual matters, including gender?

- Sexuality, sex, and relationships are integral parts of adolescent health and development.
- Gender is part of every patient and should be affirmed as part of patient-centered primary care.
- Lesbian, gay, bisexual, transgender (LGBT) youth face physical, mental, and emotional health disparities compared with their heterosexual peers.

[a] Division of Child & Adolescent Health, Columbia University Medical Center, Columbia University College of Physicians and Surgeons, 622 West 168th Street, VC4-417, New York, NY 10032, USA; [b] Division of Education, Research and Training, Physicians for Reproductive Health, 55 West 39th Street, Suite 1001, New York, NY 10018, USA; [c] Department of Pediatrics, Center for Community and Health Education, Columbia University Medical Center, New York, NY 10032, USA; [d] Department of Population and Family Health, Center for Community and Health Education, Columbia University Medical Center, 60 Haven Avenue, Level B-3, Room 308, New York, NY 10032, USA
* Corresponding author.
E-mail address: Bp35@columbia.edu

Pediatr Clin N Am 64 (2017) 291–304
http://dx.doi.org/10.1016/j.pcl.2016.11.001
0031-3955/17/© 2016 Elsevier Inc. All rights reserved.
pediatric.theclinics.com

Sexuality is an integral part of adolescent health and development and should be assessed routinely at every patient visit. Sexuality development lies on a continuum along which young people move in the context of relationships and is a healthy, natural part of life. Adolescents engage in relationships that may include a variety of sexual activities, and pediatricians play a pivotal role in supporting youth to actively participate in decision making around safe, positive sexual behaviors and practices, including abstinence if that is their choice.

Expanding social relationships and friendships is part of adolescent development. Sexual activity may be a natural and healthy outgrowth of some relationships. Healthy relationships include elements of partner support, honesty, kindness, openness, encouragement, and respect of individual space and time. In contrast, unhealthy relationships occur if a partner is overly jealous, demanding, controlling, or shaming, or if he or she physically and/or sexually hurts, humiliates, or threatens the other person.[1]

According to the 2015 Youth Risk Behavior Surveillance (YRBS), 41% of high school students report having sexual intercourse and 30% report having sexual intercourse with at least one person during the 3 months before the survey.[2] Some of these encounters were consensual, whereas others were not. YRBS found that 10% of high school students reported that the person whom they were dating deliberately hurt them physically; 11% said that they were forced to perform sexual acts that they did not want to do, and 7% said that they were physically forced to have sexual intercourse.

Adolescent relationship abuse is common and can take many forms, including emotional/mental abuse, physical abuse, sexual abuse, reproductive coercion, cyber abuse, harassment, isolation, threats, and controlling jealousy (see Elizabeth Miller's article, "Prevention and Intervention for Dating Violence in Adolescents," in this issue).

Pediatricians and other health care providers have an essential role to assess and provide routine education about healthy relationships and identify young people experiencing relationship abuse and intimate partner violence (IPV). Simply acknowledging relationship abuse, validating feelings, and providing support without judgment can create trusting relationships with patients so they feel comfortable and safe discussing these topics.

Pediatricians are uniquely positioned to talk to adolescents about sex, sexuality, and relationships as essential caregivers in their young lives. Even before adolescence begins, pediatricians have both the opportunity and the responsibility to initiate conversations about sexual matters (**Table 1**). Health care provider discomfort and lack of formal medical training for primary care providers on how to talk to adolescents about sexuality are 2 barriers to having these conversations.[3,4] Fortunately, the more one practices initiating and having these discussions, the more comfortable one becomes.

Starting these conversations early, with confidentiality pre-established, will ultimately equip adolescent patients with the knowledge and skills to make healthy decisions about their own sexual lives. Furthermore, building trust and rapport with adolescent patients helps them feel more comfortable, better prepared, and empowered to speak with future health care providers about their sexuality and sexual experiences as they enter young adulthood and beyond.

Major medical organizations, including the American Academy of Pediatrics (AAP), the American Medical Association, and the Society for Adolescent Health and Medicine, recommend that health care providers counsel and educate all adolescents about sexual matters and sexual decision making.[5,6] The 2016 AAP Clinical Report on Sexuality Education for Children and Adolescents provides specific clinical

		Female, Male, Transgender, Gender Nonconforming,
Gender Identity	**How One Self-Identifies; the Understanding of One's Self**	**Genderqueer, Nonbinary, Gender Fluid, Cisgender**
Gender expression	The way in which one acts, presents themselves, and communicates their gender identity to the outside world	May fall in line with social constructs of feminine, masculine, both, or along the spectrum
Sexual identity (sexual orientation identity)	Sexual concept of one's self that is based on feelings, attractions, and desires	Lesbian, gay, bisexual, transgender, queer/ questioning, straight, asexual, pansexual
Sexual orientation	Romantic or sexual attraction to persons of the same gender, opposite gender, all or other genders	
Pansexual	Fluid sexual attraction to people of any sex or gender	
Transgender	A person whose gender identity differs from their biological/natal sex and conventional notions of gender	FTM/transman (assigned female at birth but identifies as male) MTF/transwoman (assigned male at birth but identifies as female)
Gender nonconforming/ genderqueer/gender fluid/nonbinary	A person who views his/her gender on a spectrum rather than fitting into society's binary categories of male/ female	
Cisgender	A person whose gender identity conforms to the cultural notions of gender and the biological sex they were assigned at birth	
Queer	An umbrella term that may include the entire LGBT community and also people who fit outside social norms of sexual identity and gender expression; emphasizes fluid and experience-based identities and attractions	

Table 1
Definition of terms

Adapted from Hyderi A, Angel J, Madison M, et al. Transgender patients: providing sensitive care. J Fam Pract 2016;(65)7:450–61.

guidelines for pediatricians to both initiate conversations about sex and sexuality and discuss topics, including confidentiality, gender, sexual identity, healthy relationships and IPV, sexual pleasure, empowerment, and responsibility.[7]

Unfortunately, studies show that pediatricians do not routinely initiate talks about sexual matters, and when the topic is raised, discussions are brief and incomplete.

One observational study found that among 253 adolescents surveyed, one-third reported no discussion of sexual issues at annual visits, and when the discussion did
occur, it only lasted 36 seconds.[8] Another study of AAP members found that although
most pediatricians discussed sexual activity at preventive care visits, they rarely or
never discussed sexual identity/homosexuality.[9] This finding is especially troubling
when LGBT youth face numerous physical, mental, and emotional health disparities
compared with heterosexual youth.

Thirty to 40% of LGBT youth in the United States are homeless, and sexual minority
homeless youth have increased lifetime sexual partners, higher rates of sexually transmitted infections (STIs), and younger ages of sexual initiation.[10] A nationally representative sample found that almost one-quarter of adolescents in same-sex relationships
reported some type of IPV and those who identify as transgender experience higher
rates of IPV than both heterosexual and other LGB communities.[11] Findings from a
nationwide school survey found that LGBT youth reported increased risk of bullying
and physical/verbal harassment in the past year due to sexual orientation.[12] Bisexual
and lesbian female adolescents are at greater risk for earlier age at heterosexual
debut, more sexual partners, forced sex by male partner, unintended pregnancy,
and STIs.[13–15] Adolescents who identify as Lesbian, Gay or Bisexual also report higher
rates of depression, anxiety, suicidal thoughts, and self-harm.[16]

Although many LGBT youth are disproportionately affected by risk-taking behaviors, most grow up healthy and lead happy, productive lives. For LGBT youth,
adolescence is a developmental phase in which many physical, emotional, social,
and sexual changes take place, similarly to heterosexual youth. However, for
many sexual minority youth, these changes are more challenging and difficult
because of family disapproval, societal and internalized homophobia, and discrimi-
natory treatment in health care settings.[17] To overcome stress created by stigmatization, many LGBT youth develop and possess remarkable strength and self-
determination.[18]

*How can pediatricians help mitigate lesbian, gay, bisexual, transgender youth health
disparities?*

- Initiate discussions about gender and sexual identity
- Use inclusive, nonjudgmental language to normalize diversities in identities, at-
  tractions, and behaviors
- Provide affirming support and resources as needed

When asked questions about sexual orientation and gender identity (SOGI) by their
providers, most heterosexual and LGBT patients in primary care settings answered
them, said they would respond to such questions in the future, and expressed positive
support for the importance of asking these questions.[19] Ideally, pediatricians and
other health care providers should ask all adolescent patients standardized SOGI
questions as part of routine care. Most youth find the questions both acceptable
and important for their medical provider to know. Furthermore, most LGBT respon-
dents said the survey questions allowed them to accurately document their SOGI,
which allows providers to make a better assessment of the patient's health and potential risk factors.

In order to have inclusive conversations with all adolescent patients, it is best to use
gender-neutral language and avoid assumptions about gender identity, sexual attractions, and sexual orientation identity. One study examining language used by physicians talking with adolescents about sexuality found that inclusive talk rarely
occurred (3.3%), while noninclusive language was predominant.[20] Health care providers in these primary care clinics often assumed heterosexuality and heterosexual

sexual behaviors or more indirectly framed the talk as heterosexual. Sexual minority adolescents are prone to feeling shame and isolation when health care providers fail to use inclusive language or make assumptions about their sexuality. In qualitative interviews, those participants who identified as bisexual, gay, or pansexual reported that being asked, "How is your girlfriend/boyfriend?" as if they were heterosexual, made them feel unaccepted by their health care provider.[21]

SUMMARY

Clinicians can best serve their patients and their patients' families by becoming adept at initiating confidential and developmentally appropriate discussions about sexuality with all adolescents. Although adolescents' physical, psychosocial, emotional, and cognitive stages of development interact, they can often be discordant (**Fig. 1**). It is useful to consider this discordance as health care providers decide how to thoughtfully craft sensitive questions about sex and sexuality. Adolescents' physical changes associated with puberty, the timing of these changes, and the cognitive capacity of adolescents strongly impact their social and emotional functioning. In addition, adolescents' brains are still developing, and there is a biologic basis for increased risk taking, shortsightedness, and impulsivity often seen during adolescence.[22] Health care providers should not assume that physically mature adolescents are as cognitively mature as young adults and should adapt how they speak with adolescents to avoid missing opportunities to engage them in a developmentally appropriate manner rather than an "age-appropriate" manner.

OBTAINING THE SEXUAL HISTORY

One way of obtaining a sexual history is by using the HEEADSSS acronym.[23] This approach assesses *H*ome environment, *E*ducation and *E*mployment, *E*ating, peer-related and other *A*ctivities (including hobbies and interests), *D*rug use, *D*epression, *S*uicidality, *S*exuality, *S*afety, and *S*pirituality/Strengths. A benefit of this approach it that it begins by asking adolescents about less sensitive topics, thus affording an

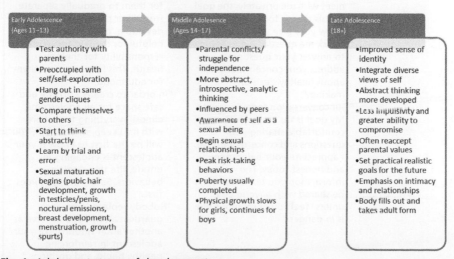

Early Adolescence (Ages 11–13)	Middle Adolescence (Ages 14–17)	Late Adolescence (18+)
•Test authority with parents •Preoccupied with self/self-exploration •Hang out in same gender cliques •Compare themselves to others •Start to think abstractly •Learn by trial and error •Sexual maturation begins (pubic hair development, growth in testicles/penis, nocturnal emissions, breast development, menstruation, growth spurts)	•Parental conflicts/ struggle for independence •More abstract, introspective, analytic thinking •Influenced by peers •Awareness of self as a sexual being •Begin sexual relationships •Peak risk-taking behaviors •Puberty usually completed •Physical growth slows for girls, continues for boys	•Improved sense of identity •Integrate diverse views of self •Abstract thinking more developed •Less impulsivity and greater ability to compromise •Often reaccept parental values •Set practical realistic goals for the future •Emphasis on intimacy and relationships •Body fills out and takes adult form

Fig. 1. Adolescent stages of development.

opportunity for health care providers to build rapport before asking more sensitive questions about sex and sexuality as well as mental health and substance use.

Health care providers should aim to create a safe, confidential, nonjudgmental space where adolescents learn about "sexual matters," discuss concerns, ask questions related to sex and sexuality, and find support for healthy development. For some adolescents, a visit with a health care provider presents the sole opportunity to discuss this important part of their lives. Pediatricians and other health care providers can be a resource to address patients' and parents' questions and concerns about sexual matters. Although it might seem like the annual physical is the only time to address these matters, realistically, almost all adolescent visits provide an opportunity to discuss sexual matters (**Table 2**).

Because health care providers often see adolescents who are minors, it is important to know state laws related to minors' rights to consent to health care services and

Table 2
How to approach the confidential visit

	Discussing Confidentiality with Youth	Discussing Confidentiality with Parents/Caregivers
Useful tips	• Explain limits to privacy and confidential parts of the visit	• Explain parameters of confidentiality/office policy • Listen to concerns, repeat back, assure you will address their concerns • Thank them and escort them to the waiting area • Invite them back before wrap up • Validate feelings if they feel uncomfortable leaving the room • Defer private visit for future, if appropriate
Helpful phrases	"At every visit, all of my patients are offered the opportunity to meet with me privately; the goal of this time is for me to get to know you, give you a chance to ask me questions, and for me to answer your questions, address your concerns, and talk about healthy decision-making." "Our conversation today is private. My goal is for you to feel comfortable sharing your questions and concerns with me. I appreciate your being open and honest today. The information you tell me will not be shared with anyone else unless I feel you or someone else is in danger."	"As adolescents grow up, it is developmentally appropriate for them to gradually separate from their parents and begin to develop a 'private self.' It is also helpful for them to begin taking responsibility for their own health. This helps prepare them for adulthood." "In order to create a private and safe space for all adolescents, almost everything they share with me I keep confidential. You will be the first to know if your adolescent is engaging in unsafe, life threatening behaviors. Safety always comes first." "Nobody replaces a parent/guardian and I hope to serve as another adult resource for your adolescent in reinforcing healthy habits and decisions."

the limits of confidentiality. (See here for the most current state laws: https://www.guttmacher.org/sites/default/files/pdfs/spibs/spib_OMCL.pdf.)

Once health care providers are acquainted with state laws, they should review the parameters of confidentiality with both adolescents and their parents or guardians at the start of every visit. Reviewing the parameters of confidentiality will clarify and set expectations for the adolescent's visit and lessen the likelihood of misunderstandings later if a parent or guardian requests confidential information. It is helpful to confirm that confidential information that is transcribed in the history about sex and sexuality will be removed should the parent request the medical records. This policy needs to be explained to the staff members who are responsible for responding to requests for medical records because such individuals are often clerical staff members and not clinicians. In addition, if a confidential prescription is given to a minor, it is useful to check with the insurance company that this will not be disclosed to the parent. Should the adolescent and/or parent or guardian object to the adolescent being seen alone, do not force the issue and be flexible. The goal of every visit is to continue building rapport and a trusting relationship with the adolescent and his/her family, which includes respecting their choices. However, in reality, many parents are grateful that their teenage daughter or son has a trusted health care provider who cares for them.

Physicians for Reproductive Health have an Adolescent Reproductive and Sexual Health Education Program (ARSHEP) that provides standardized case videos and facilitation guides intended to illustrate how pediatricians and other health care providers can best communicate with adolescent patients about sexual matters.

The video, "Asking a Parent to Step Out," demonstrates how a provider may ask a parent to leave the room to allow for one-on-one time with an adolescent patient (Video 1).

Certain best practices help establish rapport and trust with adolescents (**Fig. 2**). Of course, an adolescent also has to be willing to participate in a dialogue and answer personal questions. It is best to first normalize questions by stating that these are topics you discuss with all adolescents. Then ask permission to open up a conversation about sex and state that the purpose of knowing this information is to deliver personalized health care and answer any questions. If an adolescent says "OK" but

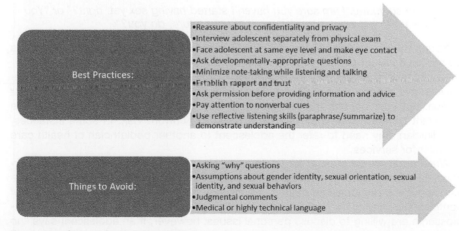

Best Practices:
- Reassure about confidentiality and privacy
- Interview adolescent separately from physical exam
- Face adolescent at same eye level and make eye contact
- Ask developmentally-appropriate questions
- Minimize note-taking while listening and talking
- Establish rapport and trust
- Ask permission before providing information and advice
- Pay attention to nonverbal cues
- Use reflective listening skills (paraphrase/summarize) to demonstrate understanding

Things to Avoid:
- Asking "why" questions
- Assumptions about gender identity, sexual orientation, sexual identity, and sexual behaviors
- Judgmental comments
- Medical or highly technical language

Fig. 2. Tips for conducting the interview.

looks uncomfortable, it is helpful to acknowledge what you see; when an adolescent's discomfort goes unacknowledged, the conversation may come to a halt or not yield an accurate history.

Suggestions for what to say include the following:

"Talking about sex may be uncomfortable and awkward for many people. If you would like, we can move on and discuss something else. I am asking for this information so I can provide you with the best health care and you are the best judge about what you do and do not want to talk about at this visit." As the conversation unfolds, it is also useful to summarize what you have heard. This summarization shows that you are listening and provides an opportunity for the adolescent to correct any misperceptions.

It is important to recognize that adolescents are also very perceptive of their provider's nonverbal cues and body language. Young people may feel judged if they are talking about their sexual attractions, experiences, or identities and their pediatrician looks confused or shocked. Adolescents can sense physician discomfort through a change in voice patterns, stammering, facial expressions, and tone of voice as was documented in a recent study that interviewed sexual minority and majority adolescents about their experiences talking about sexuality with health care providers.[18] In a concerted effort to appear comfortable and relaxed with adolescents when discussing sex and sexuality, it is essential that clinicians be aware of their nonverbal and verbal behaviors and be mindful of certain phrases and language that may appear to be judgmental and interrogative.

There are some approaches to interviewing adolescents that can be alienating and are best to avoid.

Assumptions

Avoid assumptions about gender identity, sexual orientation, sexual identity, and sexual behaviors. High functioning adolescents can engage in risk-taking sexual behaviors and risk-taking adolescents have numerous strengths; find those strengths and applaud them.

Judgment

Avoid judgmental comments, such as:

"You are so young. I am sure you haven't started having sex yet, right?" or *"You don't want to get pregnant now and hurt your future, do you?"*

Asking "why" can also be perceived as judgmental. Even adult patients sometimes do not have insight behind their behaviors and motivations.

Health care providers may have negative reactions to adolescents' beliefs and behaviors. It is important to realize that the adolescent patient is not you, your daughter or son, but your patient. If a clinician finds himself/herself feeling judgmental, it is important to reconsider what can be done at the current visit. In some instances, the clinician may need to refer the adolescent to another pediatrician or health care provider for services.

When adolescents present for health care, they may not expect to be asked personal questions, let alone questions about sexual matters. When beginning a discussion about any personal information, it is always useful to reinforce the parameters of confidentiality and to frame the reason for asking these questions (**Table 3**). Most adolescents are willing to discuss personal issues; however, if an adolescent says "no thanks," you can explore further or honor the request to not discuss the topic and

Table 3 Starting the conversation	
	Introducing Questions About Sexual Matters
Questioning style	• Use open-ended questions when possible • Highlight patients' strengths • Applaud patients' willingness to share personal information honestly
Helpful scripts	"I see you are here for a sports physical and I would like to get to know you better by asking you questions about things you do outside of this office. I welcome everyone into my practice and, unless you tell me that you are unsafe, at risk of hurting yourself or someone else, everything we discuss I will keep confidential. Some of the questions I am going to ask you are personal and some young people might find them embarrassing. I ask these questions of every young person I see so I can offer you my best care and advice that is specific for you." "When it comes to matters related to sex, there is a wide spectrum of choices adolescents make and questions that they may have. I respect ALL choices that my patients make and am always happy to answer any questions. Is it OK with you for us to discuss these matters?" "It is my goal to help you feel comfortable sharing sensitive and personal information with me. I do not make judgments. I respect you and appreciate your thoughts, feelings, and experiences that you share with me."

defer until the next visit. When you respect an adolescent's choice, you help build a therapeutic, respectful relationship.

Two versions of a how to initiate conversations on sexual matters during a sports physical examination are presented in ARSHEP case videos (Videos 2 and 3). Each clip shows different techniques for talking about sex and sexuality. Neither one is the "correct" way, but rather presents items that the provider does well and areas to improve in order to facilitate discussion.

Adolescents often develop romantic and sexual relationships with people of all genders as a part of exploring their own sexuality. Development of gender identity and sexual identity are all a part of healthy development; the array of possible combinations is limitless and complex and can be fluid and change over time. Sometimes, gender identity and expression line up with traditional social constructs of masculine and feminine; other times they do not. Adolescents' cultural, developmental, and personal factors may affect their ability to accept or express their feelings of physical and emotional attraction toward others [24] Frequently, sexual orientation and sexual identity are concordant, but this is not always the case. For example, a young man may feel sexually attracted to and even have sexual intercourse with women and at the same time identify as "gay."

There are few places where adolescents can address questions and concerns related to sex and gender: the health care provider's office should be one of these. By comfortably discussing these topics, health care providers can help adolescents gain more insight into themselves and reinforce the diversity of gender identity, gender expression, sexual identity, and sexual attraction (**Table 4**).

By gaining an understanding about an adolescent's relationships, health care providers can best assess how to counsel each patient. To put adolescents at ease and promote honest answers, open conversations with a statement like: "If you agree, in

Table 4
Interviewing adolescents about gender identity and sexual attraction/sexual identity

	Gender Identity	Sexual Attraction/Sexual Identity
Tips	Ask all adolescent patients	Ask all adolescent patients
Sample questions	The name on your chart is _____. What would you like me to call you? What is your preferred name?	"Do you have crushes? If yes, on boys, girls, both or people of other genders?"
	What gender pronouns do you prefer I use when I talk with you? He or she? His or her? Or some other pronoun like them, their, they?	"Some young people your age find themselves attracted to boys, girls, both, or other genders and some are not yet sure. This is completely natural and can change over time. Who do you find yourself sexually attracted to? How comfortable are you with your feelings of attraction?"
	"When people are born, they are assigned a gender, like male or female. Sometimes on the inside a person can feel differently than their assigned gender and, if a person feels this, it is completely natural. How much does your inside gender and assigned gender match? How comfortable are you with your gender?"	"What is your understanding of the meaning of sexual identity (also called sexual orientation identity)? What do you consider your sexual identity to be? Gay, straight, bisexual, asexual, queer, or another?"
	"Do you ever feel confused about your gender?"	
	If yes, "Is there someone who you can talk to about these feelings?"	
	"Do your parents know that you feel more like a female inside (for the male)? How did they respond to learning about this?"	

an effort to get to know you better, I will ask you about your relationships. I am not here to judge you and I welcome everyone and all choices they make." When adolescents agree to talk about relationships, ask questions using gender-neutral language such as "partners" rather than "boyfriend" or "girlfriend" to both reinforce the above comment and avoid making any assumptions based on physical presentation. Reviewing relationships at all visits is advised because relationships, choice of partners, gender of partners, and risk for sexual abuse or coercion may change over time (**Table 5**).

Generally, in speaking with the younger, less mature adolescents, it is best to begin by asking about kissing and touching and read body language as you bring up the topic and explore it. It is often less threatening to ask about adolescents' friends' activities first (**Table 6**). Adolescents may feel embarrassed or self-conscious if they are not yet having sex, especially if their peers are. Take this opportunity to affirm their healthy decision to be abstinent, emphasize that this choice is up to them, offer them permission to change their minds, and welcome them back to discuss sexual decision making with you at any time. Health care providers should not assume that all older adolescents are engaging in sexual behaviors; many choose to postpone such activities.

Open-ended questions are the most effective way to elicit a comprehensive sexual history and, at the same time, there is also a role for concrete, directive and

Table 5
Assessing the health of the relationship and partner history

	Partner History	Assessing the Health of the Relationship/Abuse/Coercion
Tips	Use gender-neutral language	Use gender-neutral language
Sample questions	"Tell me about your past and current sexual partners." "How many lifetime partners have you had oral, anal, or vaginal sex with?" "Has someone ever touched your penis/vagina?" Have you ever touched someone's penis/vagina? "How old were you when you first engaged in the above activities?"	"Tell me what a healthy relationship looks like to you." "Tell me about some of the nice and caring things that your partner does for you." "How did you and your partner decide to have sex?" "Is your partner much older/younger than you?" "How do you feel when you are with your partner?" "Sometimes people are treated or touched in a way that they don't like or are forced to do sexual things they don't want to do. Has anyone ever touched you in a sexual way that you did not like or forced you to do anything sexual?" If yes, "Tell me about that."" "You seem to really want to end this relationship because you feel pressure from your partner to begin/keep having sex and you seem unsure about how to accomplish that. What are some ways you might deal with this situation?"

close-ended questions. Once the health care provider has determined that an adolescent has engaged in oral, vaginal, or anal sex, ask questions to assess age of onset, behavior-specific questions about types of sexual behaviors, partner gender or genders, and number of partners. Taking the opportunity to reinforce that the enjoyable parts of sex are completely *natural* and *positive* is always valuable because it helps adolescents feel supported in the choices they make (see **Table 6**).

WHAT NEXT? WHAT TO DO WITH THE SEXUAL HISTORY

Adolescents often have numerous concerns, questions, and other health issues to address at any visit. Not every issue needs to be addressed at one visit. If an adolescent is engaging in multiple unhealthy behaviors and is interested in change, the adolescent with the health care provider can choose 1 or 2 behaviors to work on at a time. The clinician can discuss concrete changes that the adolescent thinks are feasible and then help the adolescent think through how to implement the plan. Schedule an early follow-up visit to review how things are progressing and decide if changes are necessary. For health care providers who would rather refer to another professional for ongoing management, it is imperative to know local referral sources, for example, mental health providers, social workers, domestic violence advocates, or adolescent medicine specialists within the institution or community (**Table 7**).

Table 6
Asking about sexual behaviors, sexual function, and pleasure/satisfaction

Development Stage	Sexual Behaviors	Sexual Function and Sexual Pleasure/Satisfaction
Early adolescence	"As young people grow up, some become curious and interested in kissing, touching and some may even become curious about and interested in other sexual behaviors. What are your thoughts, interests, or experiences with any of these activities?" "Tell me about your friends." "What sort of things do you and your friends do together?" "Have any of your friends begun kissing/touching?"	"Many young people have questions about sex including about erections and ejaculating or cumming, vaginal lubrication or wetness, foreplay, and others have questions about their bodies or other general questions. What questions do you have?"
Middle adolescence	"Choosing to wait to have sex is a very healthy choice and sometimes people change their minds. When you have questions about sex, or when you decide that this is something you are considering, please come in to see me so we can have a confidential discussion about how you can keep yourself safe." "Tell me about when you started to participate in different sexual behaviors like touching a person's genitals (like their penis or vagina) or having your genitals touched, or having, oral, vaginal, or anal sex."	"Some young people are having sex and are enjoying it while others are not or may not be feeling pleasure or having orgasms. Please share with me your experiences with sexual satisfaction or pleasure." "Some young people choose alternatives to sex such as masturbation which is a healthy normal choice. Would you like to discuss this in more detail? Feel free to tell me what you would like to discuss or what questions you might have."
Later adolescence	"Many young people engage in a variety of sexual behaviors, like oral, vaginal, and anal sex. Have you engaged in any of these behaviors?" "It is completely normal for some young people to feel curiosity about different types of sexual exploration. Some choose to have sexual behaviors with males, females, both, and/or other genders. Tell me about the choices you have made."	"Do you ever have pain when you have sex or questions about your sexual functioning?" "What does sexual satisfaction mean to you?" "If you are not sexually satisfied, what do you think would need to change to improve your satisfaction?" "How comfortable are you talking with your partner about sexual satisfaction and pleasure?" "Tell me about some of the things your partner does to ensure your sexual satisfaction?" Is there anything about your relationship with your partner that you wish that you could change?

Table 7 Resources	
Physicians for Reproductive Health, Adolescent Reproductive and Sexual Health Education Program (ARSHEP)	https://prh.org/teen-reproductive-health/arshep-explained/
Family Acceptance Project	familyproject.sfsu.edu
Parents and Friends of Lesbians and Gays	www.pflag.org
Centers for Disease Control LGBT Fact Sheet & Resource	cdc.gov/lgbthealth/transgender.htm
National Center for Transgender Equality	www.transequality.org
Guttmacher Institute	https://www.guttmacher.org/state-policy/explore/overview-minors-consent-law
Futures Without Violence	FuturesWithoutViolence.org

Every patient visit is an opportunity to obtain a sexual history from an adolescent and discuss sexual matters. With practice, these interviews become more comfortable; with increasing comfort, these conversations can occur quickly and efficiently. By eliciting adolescents' questions, concerns, and feelings about sexual matters, pediatricians and other health care providers can reinforce natural, positive sexual development and guide adolescents toward healthy lifestyles.

SUPPLEMENTARY DATA

Supplementary video related to this article can be found at http://dx.doi.org/10.1016/j.pcl.2016.11.001.

REFERENCES

1. Miller E, Catalozzi M. Promoting healthy relationships & responding to adolescent relationship abuse: ARA PART I. 2016. Available at: http://www.nypath.org/ekp1/nypath/public/archived-webinars.html. Accessed August 9, 2016.
2. Centers for Disease Control and Prevention. 2015. Youth Risk Behavior Survey Data. Available at: www.cdc.gov/yrbs. Accessed August 9, 2016.
3. Boekeloo B. Will you ask? Will they tell you? Are you ready to hear and respond?: barriers to physician-adolescent discussion about sexuality. JAMA Pediatr 2014; 168(2):111–3.
4. CGME Program Requirements for Graduate Medical Education in Pediatrics. 2016. Available at: https://www.acgme.org/Portals/0/PFAssets/ProgramRequirements/320_pediatrics_2016.pdf. Accessed August 9, 2016.
5. Burke P, Coles M, Meglio G, et al. Sexual and reproductive health care: a position paper of the society for adolescent health and medicine. J Adolesc Health 2014; 54:491–6.
6. American Medical Association. Guidelines for adolescent prevention services (GAPS). Chicago: American Medical Association; 1997.
7. Breuner C, Mattson G. AAP Committee on adolescence, AAP Committee on Psychosocial Aspects of Child and Family Health. Sexuality education for children and adolescents. Pediatrics 2016;138(2):e20161348.
8. Alexander S, Fortenberry J, Pollak K, et al. Sexuality talk during adolescent health maintenance visits. JAMA Pediatr 2014;168(2):163–9.
9. Henry-Reid L, O'Connor K, Klein J, et al. Current pediatrician practices in identifying high-risk behaviors of adolescents. Pediatrics 2010;125(4):e741–7.

10. McBride D. Homelessness and health care disparities among lesbian, gay, bisexual, and transgender youth. J Pediatr Nurs 2012;27(2):177–9.
11. Halpern C, Young M, Waller M, et al. Prevalence of partner violence in same-sex romantic and sexual relationships in a national sample of adolescents. J Adolesc Health 2004;35(2):124–31.
12. Kosciw J, Greytak E, Bartkiewicz M, et al. The 2011 National School Climate Survey: the experiences of lesbian, gay, bisexual and transgender youth in our nation's schools. New York: GLSEN; 2012.
13. Tornello S, Riskind R, Patterson C. Sexual orientation and sexual and reproductive health among adolescent young women in the United States. J Adolesc Health 2014;54(2):160–8.
14. Marrazzo J, Koutsky L, Kiviat N, et al. Papanicolaou test screening and prevalence of genital human papillomavirus among women who have sex with women. Am J Public Health 2001;91:947–52.
15. Lindley L, Walsemann K. Sexual orientation and risk of pregnancy among New York City high-school students. Am J Public Health 2015;105(7):1379–86.
16. Shearer A, Herres J, Kodish T, et al. Differences in mental health symptoms across lesbian, gay, bisexual, and questioning youth in primary care settings. J Adolesc Health 2016;59:38–43.
17. Lambda Legal. When health care isn't caring: Lambda legal's survey of discrimination against LGBT people and people with HIV. 2010. Available at: www.lambdalegal.org/health-care-report. Accessed August 9, 2016.
18. Garofalo R, Katz E. Health care issues of gay and lesbian youth. Curr Opin Pediatr 2001;13:298–302.
19. Cahill S, Singal R, Grasso C, et al. Do ask, do tell: high levels of acceptability by patients of routine collection of sexual orientation and gender identity data in four diverse American community health centers. PLoS One 2014;9(9):e107104.
20. Alexander S, Fortenberry J, Pollak K, et al. Physicians use of inclusive sexual orientation language during teenage annual visits. LGBT Health 2014;1(4):283–91.
21. Fuzzell L, Fedesco HN, Alexander SC, et al. "I just think that doctors need to ask more questions": sexual minority and majority adolescents' experiences talking about sexuality with healthcare providers. Patient Educ Couns 2016;99(9):1467–72.
22. Hazen E, Schlozman S, Beresin E. Adolescent psychological development: a review. Pediatr Rev 2008;29(5):161–7.
23. Klein D, Goldenring J, Adelman W. HEEADSSS 3.0: the psychosocial interview for adolescents updated for a new century fueled by media. Contemp Pediatr 2014;31:16–28.
24. Frankowski B. Sexual orientation and adolescents. Pediatrics 2004;113:1827–32.

Talking to Parents About Adolescent Sexuality

Amie M. Ashcraft, PhD, MPH[a],*, Pamela J. Murray, MD, MHP[b]

KEYWORDS

- Adolescent • Sexuality • Communication • Parent • Prevention

KEY POINTS

- Parents are an influential source of information about sexuality to their adolescents and have the ability to shape these values and behaviors.
- Parents should communicate comprehensive, medically accurate information to their teens.
- Parents should incorporate discussions about positive aspects of sexuality, such as pleasure, satisfaction, and intimacy, into these conversations.
- There are resources available for providers, parents, and teens for information, guidance, and support, and the major ones are highlighted here.

INTRODUCTION

The importance of parents, guardians, and other caregivers (henceforth referred to as "parents," but inclusive of the adults who function in a parenting role) in all aspects of adolescent development cannot be overstated, but their role in sexual education is crucial. Parents are the single largest influence on their adolescents' decisions about sex, and parents underestimate the impact they have on their decisions.[1] For most parents and their children, the prospect of talking about topics related to sexuality creates anxiety and apprehension, and this may lead to avoidance of discussions (**Table 1** provides a list of common sources of anxiety associated with talking about sexuality).

Parents may also delay conversations about sexuality because they are afraid of putting ideas into their child's head before they are "ready" or because they equate talking about sexuality with giving tacit permission to explore sexual behaviors. In fact, sex education and parent-child communication about sexuality are associated with delayed sexual activity and more consistent contraceptive use.[2–4] Conversations with parents

The authors have nothing to disclose.
[a] Department of Pediatrics, West Virginia University School of Medicine, Box 9216, Morgantown, WV 26506, USA; [b] Department of Pediatrics, West Virginia University School of Medicine, Box 9214, Morgantown, WV 26506, USA
* Corresponding author.
E-mail address: amashcraft@hsc.wvu.edu

Table 1 Sources of anxiety for parents and teens when discussing sexuality	
Sources of Anxiety for Parents	**Sources of Anxiety for Teens**
Real or perceived ignorance • Not knowing the answers • Not knowing the correct language to use/ sounding crude • Being wrong or corrected • Having different answers than other parent or adult	Real or perceived ignorance • Not knowing the correct language to use/ sounding crude • Not knowing the right questions to ask • Being wrong or corrected
Saying too much • Providing more information than your child is ready for • Revealing too much personal information (TMI) • Revealing family secrets • Disclosure of abuse (of self or another)	Saying too much • Revealing sexual thoughts or behaviors to the parent that might elicit criticism or punishment • Disclosure of abuse (of self or another)
Fear of difficult questions • About how babies are made • About contraception, fertility, abortion, pregnancy, and so forth • About parent's own adolescent behaviors or adult sexuality • About prior relationships, separation, divorce, or death • About abuse experiences • About the sexuality spectrum	Fear of difficult questions • Questions about current sexual behavior • Questions about abuse • Questions about the sexuality spectrum
Finding out something unknown about child • Is already sexually active, uses contraception, or had an abortion • Has experienced abuse or vulnerability to abuse • Is LGBTQIA • Has been exposed to pornography • Has "sexted" or sent explicit language or photos via social media	Finding out something unknown about parent • About their current or past sex life • A negative family secret • Disclosure of abuse
Fear of teen's reaction/perception • Sounding stupid • Sounding "old-fashioned" or out of touch • Teen will not be open to the conversation/ topic • Disclosure of abuse	Fear of parent's reaction/perception • Sounding stupid • Parent will not be open to the conversation/topic • Asking something that shocks, offends, or angers the parent • Asking something the parent refuses to answer • Disclosure of abuse
Discomfort with topic • Embarrassment • Shame • Fear	Discomfort with topic • Embarrassment • Shame • Fear

have the potential to become the benchmarks against which teens measure other information about sexuality and serve as a buffer against early sexual activity.

Unfortunately, in many instances, "sex talks" between parents and their children are less than optimal. Parents tend to exclude positive topics associated with sexuality, such as pleasure, love, and healthy relationships, in favor of negative topics and warnings. These conversations lacking positive topics associated with sexuality, pregnancy, sexually transmitted infections (STIs), and abuse and exploitation. Parental guidance is needed as adolescents develop, but parents need to have accurate and complete information from medically accurate resources to share with their teens. The purpose of this article is to provide an overview of the best practices, specific tips, and resources that health care providers can use to empower parents.

Parents Talking with Adolescents About Sexuality: Best Practices

This article is an overview of currently understood best practices related to talking to adolescents about sexuality within the context of contemporary knowledge and broad cultural norms. For the sake of brevity, the authors describe the best practices in relation to major topics in sexuality.

Talking about sexuality, in general

The groundwork for communication about sexuality is laid in early childhood and takes place over the course of many interactions and "teachable moments"—opportunities that arise to start a conversation or provide information about a topic—as opposed to one "big talk" about "the birds and the bees." Regular and ongoing discussions support and reinforce concepts addressed in earlier conversations and increase the likelihood the child will encode the content to memory and have it cognitively accessible later. Some parents and teens may have discussed sexuality in the past but have not done so recently. An absence of conversation may be an indicator that it is time for parents to check in with their teen.

When it comes to conversations about sexuality, parents may have different ideas about what constitutes a "conversation" than their children. Parents report more frequent communication about sex than their teens, in part because they consider a wider array of topics to be sex-related than teens, including generalized warnings indirectly related to sex, such as "Stay away from boys. Period."[5] Some parents may defer to these blanket warnings because they do not know where to begin or how to be more specific. In order to prepare parents for what to expect and where to start, **Table 2** highlights what children and adolescents tend to know and ask about concerning sexuality across their development. **Box 1** suggests teachable moments when parents may want to consider having a conversation related to sexuality.

Topics covered when talking about sexuality

Many parents focus on providing factual and mechanical information about sex and neglect discussion of emotions, sexual pleasure, and values. There is likely a fear that portraying sex in too positive a light may entice and encourage experimentation. Parents may need help understanding that conversations about sexuality can be factual and sex positive while simultaneously communicating boundaries and values. These conversations are opportune times for parents to relate their values and expectations in relation to their child's behavior. For example, "If you have sex, we believe it is important to use a condom for your health and safety. Condoms help prevent STIs and unintended pregnancy." When appropriate, parents may want to share decisions that they may have regretted in their own teen years and discuss how they might have handled situations differently.

Anatomy/physiology

Parents should begin teaching children age-appropriate words for body parts and their functions at an early age. There are several excellent books for children and teens

Table 2
What kids know and what questions parents can expect from their children across adolescence

Age Range	What Kids Know	Questions to Expect
7–10 y (preadolescence)	• Words for genitals, breasts • Body parts and functions (basic version) • Bathroom humor	Physical development and how they compare to others (what's "normal"). Some girls will begin puberty or menstruation at this age and should be prepared by their parents. Examples include: • What is a period? • When will I start? • When did you start? • When will my breasts grow?
11–12 y (early adolescence)	• Words for sex • Body parts and functions (expanded version) • May use sexual words even though they may not know the precise meaning • Bathroom humor and sexual humor • May have seen pornography online • Sexting	Sex education in school starts around 5th or 6th grade. Parents should allow their children to participate and continue the conversation at home. Questions may focus on the mechanics of sex and pregnancy: • What is masturbation? (self vs other) • What is oral sex? Anal sex? • Sexuality spectrum (eg, what is "gay"? How does someone know they are gay?) • How do gay people have sex? • How does a girl get pregnant? • What is an erection? Nocturnal emissions?
13–14 y (early midadolescence)	• Basic understanding of most sexual behaviors • Growing sexual vocabulary • Many have begun masturbation • Some teens will begin engaging in sexual behaviors with partners (eg, kissing, touching) • Some teens will experience love	Most girls will have begun menstruation, and most boys will be experiencing erections. Teens will have questions related to sex and pregnancy: • How old should I be when I have sex for the first time? • How old were you when you had sex for the first time? • How do I decide when to have sex with someone? • What is an orgasm? • Can women have orgasms? • Can I get pregnant the first time I have sex? • What do condoms feel like?

(continued on next page)

| Table 2 | | |
| *(continued)* | | |
Age Range	What Kids Know	Questions to Expect
15–16 y (late midadolescence)	• Most have begun masturbation • Understanding conse- quences to sexual behavior, such as pregnancy and infection/disease • Sexual behaviors with part- ners, some intercourse • Difficulty discerning love and lust	Approximately 15% of teens begin having sex by the age of 15.[5] More questions will focus on the risk of various activities for pregnancy or STIs and prevention. • Can I get an STI from kiss- ing? Oral sex? Anal sex? • How can I tell if I have an STI? • How can you tell if someone has an STI? • What is HIV/AIDS? • How effective are condoms? Birth control pills? Shots? (and so forth) • What is emergency contraception and how do I know if I need it? • How/where do I get condoms? Birth control pills? (and so forth)
17–18 + years (late adolescence)	• Difficulty discerning love and lust • Most teens have engaged in at least one sexual behavior with a partner	About 50% of teens begin having sex between the ages of 17 and 18[5] and likely experience intense physical and emotional attraction to their partners or potential partners. Questions may arise around romantic love: • How do you know if you are in love? • Were you in love the first time you had sex?

that model age-appropriate terminology (**Table 3**).[6] There is increasing evidence that using anatomically correct words—such as penis, scrotum, vagina, and vulva—is beneficial to children's early development of body confidence, self-empowerment, and safety.[7,8] Many parents feel more comfortable teaching their children generic, playful, or distracting words to identify their anatomy. There is some concern that the use of euphemisms sends the message that these parts are embarrassing, secret, or shameful. Using common names for these parts facilitates conversations about how to keep them healthy, clean, and safe. Speaking comfortably about these topics early on will help children express concerns about health, illness, relationships, sex, shaming, exploitation, or abuse in the future.

Puberty

As the child approaches the preteen years, parents should begin talking to them about puberty and what it means for their physical appearance, feelings, and reproductive ability. The "prepuberty years"—when some children begin the pubertal maturation

---

Box 1
Examples of teachable moments related to sexuality

From the mass media
- News coverage of a case related to rape, sexual abuse, and so forth
- Shared media experiences (television, movie, YouTube, music, and so forth) depicting a romantic or sexual situation, such as portrayal of 2 people going on a date, or a gay/lesbian couple, transgender people
- Portrayals of men and women in advertisements
- Portrayals of transgender people in the media
- Celebrity coverage of almost anything

From social media
- Mentions of body weight/size/judgments in pictures and picture comments (eg, thigh gaps, statements related to looking fat or skinny)
- Idealized and sexualized images
- Bullying and sexual harassment
- Posts from the "It Gets Better" campaign
- Sexting and/or other social media issues

Major life events or developments
- Pregnancy, miscarriage, birth, or adoption in the family or friends
- A friend or family member "coming out" as gay, lesbian, bisexual, transgender, and so forth
- Menarche

Everyday occurrences
- A pet giving birth or laying eggs
- Overhearing the use of sexual slurs, such as fag, whore, slut, and so forth
- Expressions of affection between people in public or semipublic places
- Family media sharing or meal conversations

---

process—begins as early as primary school. In a second grade class, it is likely that some girls have begun to develop body odor, breasts, pubic hair, and height. Changes in some boys may start in the next few grades, and understanding the process enough to be respectful and supportive of others is part of this conversation.

Masturbation

Masturbation is a frequently neglected topic because of the potential for discomfort, embarrassment, and widespread misinformation, but teens need to understand that masturbation is normal and healthy. It can provide an outlet for sexual urges that carries no risk of pregnancy or STIs. It can be self-soothing and calming. In addition to reassuring teens that masturbation is a healthy part of sexuality, parents should communicate the appropriate times and places for engagement in this behavior.

Oral sex and anal sex

Many parents do not discuss oral and anal sex specifically with their adolescents. As a result, teens are largely unaware of the risks associated with oral and anal sex. Many teens will engage in one or both of these behaviors to avoid pregnancy but inadvertently put themselves at risk for disease—especially if barrier protection is not used. Parents should educate themselves and their teens regarding barrier methods of prevention, how to use them correctly, and how to obtain them. Purchasing condoms, and keeping them in an accessible place, can be a powerful conversation opener, and in some communities is considered a normative part of parenting an adolescent.

Abstinence

Many parents want to present teens with abstinence as their *only* option when it comes to sexual behavior. Although teens have times when they are abstinent, it is

Table 3
Resources for providers, parents, and adolescents

Resource	Contact Information/Web Site	Description/Useful Features
Advocates for Youth	(202) 347–5700 AdvocatesForYouth.org	Works in both the United States and abroad to promote sexual health education and services for youth. Web site includes resources, continuing education opportunities, and curricula for sex educators
American Academy of Pediatrics (AAP)	AAP.org HealthyChildren.org BrightFutures.aap.org	Professional guidelines and standards for pediatric care. Specific useful resources: 1. Healthy Children: Contains recommendations and best practices for pediatric care. 2. Bright Futures: Provides AAP guidelines for overall adolescent physical, mental, reproductive, and social health supervision. Includes Periodicity Schedule as well as curricula and tools for adolescent health promotion and education
American Congress of Obstetricians and Gynecologists (ACOG)	ACOG.org/About-ACOG/ACOG-Departments/Adolescent-Health-Care	Information and resources for adolescent sexuality and sex education
American Sexual Health Association (ASHA)	(919) 361–8400 ASHASexualHealth.org IWannaKnow.org	Organization advocating for sexual health education and policy to promote sexual health. Web site includes especially good information for teens, including suggested questions to ask a health care provider about sex
Answer: sex ed, honestly	answer.rutgers.edu	Provides training and education to teachers and other youth-serving professionals. Web site also includes resources for parents and teens
Bedsider & Bedsider Provider (a program by The National Campaign to Prevent Teen and Unplanned Pregnancy)	Bedsider.org Providers.Bedsider.org	Bedsider: An online birth control support network that includes a hotline for free birth control information and e-mail or text reminders for birth control, appointments, prescription refills, and gonorrhea and chlamydia retests Bedsider provider: Resources to offer patients, frequently asked questions for providers, and "Shoptalk": currents events, updates, and featured resources in the world of reproductive health care practice and research

(continued on next page)

Table 3
(continued)

Resource	Contact Information/Web Site	Description/Useful Features
Boston Children's Hospital	YoungMensHealthSite.org YoungWomensHealth.org	Provides medically accurate information, educational programs, and conferences about many health topics, including sex
The Center for Sex Education (CSE)	(973) 387–5161 SexEdCenter.org	An organization within Planned Parenthood that writes and publishes resources on sex education. Includes an online bookstore (www.sexedstore.com) with books, curricula, and training manuals for sex educators and parents. CSE sells several books authored by Robie H. Harris recommended within this article
The Centers for Disease Control and Prevention (CDC)	(404) 639–3311 CDC.gov	US federal agency that works to promote health, prevention, and preparedness activities in the United States and worldwide. Includes a useful tip sheet for talking with parents about the HPV vaccine (referenced within this article) at http://www.cdc.gov/vaccines/who/teens/for-hcp.html
Center for Parent Information and Resources	ParentCenterHub.org	Information for parents and teachers about sexual education for students with disabilities, including specific disabilities, such as autism spectrum disorders, cerebral palsy, and spina bifida
Futures Without Violence	FuturesWithoutViolence.org	Organization focused on ending domestic and sexual violence. Provides free resource cards (in large quantities, if necessary) containing screening questions for IPV in adolescents
Go Ask Alice! (from Columbia University)	GoAskAlice.columbia.edu	Provides questions and answers on a variety of health topics, including sexual health. Maintains a large question and answer library and accepts new questions
IMPACT on Health and Wellness (an initiative by the Maternal Child and Health Bureau of US Department of Health and Human Services [DHHS])	Family Voices, Inc Phone (505) 872–4774 or (888) 835–5669 fv-impact.org/	Information and resources promoting maternal and child health including The Well Visit Planner—an online tool to help families prepare for their upcoming well-child visits (available in English and Spanish)

(continued on next page)

Table 3 *(continued)*		
Resource	**Contact Information/Web Site**	**Description/Useful Features**
KidsHealth (by Nemours)	KidsHealth.org	Provides health information about kids and teens that is free of "doctor speak"
The Mediatrician	http://cmch.tv/parents/askthemediatrician/	A Web site where a pediatrician offers research-based information and advice to parents about their children's media use and its implications for their health and wellness
The National Campaign to Prevent Teen And Unplanned Pregnancy	(202) 478–8500 TeenPregnancy.org	An organization providing national and state statistics on teen pregnancy, poll results, and analyses of factors affecting sex education and teen sexual behavior and contractive use. Promotes teen sexual health through initiatives such as Bedsider and Bedsider Provider
North American Society for Pediatric and Adolescent Gynecology (NASPAG)	(856) 423–3064 E-mail: hq@naspag.org NASPAG.org	Professional organization devoted to promoting research and education related to gynecologic care in youth; holds an annual meeting
Office of Adolescent Health	(240) 453–2846 http://www.hhs.gov/ash/oah/	Department within the US DHHS that funds research and interventions to reduce unplanned pregnancy and STIs in adolescents. Maintains a list of Evidence-Based Programs (EBPs) for pregnancy and STIs and a list of federal resources (tip sheets, fact sheets, treatment guidelines, and so forth) for adolescent health, including reproductive health
Parent Advocacy Coalition for Educational Rights (PACER)	(952) 838–9000 1–800–537–2237 Pacer.org	Training, information, and resource center for families of youth with disabilities—includes sexuality
PFLAG (formerly known as Parents, Families, and Friends of Lesbians and Gays)	PFLAG.org	Advocates for gay, lesbian, bisexual, and transgendered people and their families
Planned Parenthood Federation of America (PPFA)	(212) 541–7800 PlannedParenthood.org	Provider and advocate for reproductive health care and education across the United States
Scarleteen	Scarleteen.com	Highest-ranked Web site for sex education and sexuality advice; read by youth 15–25

(continued on next page)

Table 3 (continued)		
Resource	Contact Information/Web Site	Description/Useful Features
Sex, Etc.	Sexetc.org	Magazine and Web site offering sexual education and health information to teens. Includes material written by teens, forums for discussion, sexual health videos, blogs on current events, a state-by-state guide to teen rights in sex education, birth control, and health care
Sexuality Information and Education Council of the United States (SIECUS)	(212) 819–9770 siecus.org	Organization that provides policy, community action, and research updates on hot-button issues related to sexuality and sexuality education. Has a free toolkit for providers: PrEP Education for Youth-Serving Primary Care Providers Toolkit
Society for Adolescent Health and Medicine (SAHM)	AdolescentHealth.org THRIVE app	Multidisciplinary professional organization promoting adolescent health through advocacy, clinical care, health promotion, professional development, and research. Holds an annual meeting
Urban Dictionary, LLC	UrbanDictionary.com	This is "the" Web site to look up slang words and phrases. The contents are crowd sourced and continuously updated– especially sex-related slang– useful for parents trying to interpret mass media and social media their child is exposed to, such as common expressions, slang words, and acronyms
Your Child Development and Behavioral Resources	www.med.umich.edu/yourchild/	Web site for materials, resources, and useful Web sites for families of youth with disabilities— includes sexuality education resources

not an effective life-long plan. Parents may encourage abstinence and share their values around their support, but this strategy is not advised in isolation. Parents should teach that it is the only 100% effective way to avoid pregnancy and disease, but also how to protect themselves if they become sexually active. Research shows that adolescents with abstinence-only sexual education are no more likely to abstain from sex than adolescents who received no sexual education at all.[9]

Harm reduction
Most adolescents classify sexual behaviors as "safe" or "unsafe" and fail to appreciate the concept of relative risk.[10] Pediatric providers can teach parents and teens to think of sexual behaviors along a continuum from "less risky" to "very risky" and encourage

parents to suggest ways to achieve sexual pleasure with a partner that involve less risk than intercourse, such as hugging, kissing, mutual masturbation, and oral sex. Some parents may balk at the idea of encouraging these "less risky" behaviors, but providing them with a more nuanced understanding of risk minimization strategies can protect their teen's health.

Prevention
Prevention is multifaceted, and risk factors for a host of unwanted or consequential health outcomes in adolescents are interrelated. Prevention efforts come in many forms, and parents can enhance prevention of a variety of negative outcomes and enhance their child's overall health promotion by

- Increasing communication and positive family interactions;
- Being involved in their school and homework;
- Setting clear boundaries and providing consistent and caring discipline;
- Monitoring their behavior, including their activities, engagement, interests, and online participation;
- Getting to know their friends;
- Identifying teachable moments related to sex, gender, identity, sexual orientation, relationships, decision making, sexual behavior, contraception, and life goals;
- Encouraging good health practices, including diet, sleep, and exercise;
- Teaching healthy ways to cope with stress, anxiety, and negative events;
- Scheduling appointments with a pediatric provider regularly for age-appropriate care;
- Communicating about sexuality, including facts, values, and expectations;
- Educating about protections from STIs and unwanted pregnancy;
- Encouraging involvement in school and community activities;
- Engaging with schools, community programs, and faith-based organizations providing sexual health education to youth to discuss whether the information provided is comprehensive, medically accurate, and evidence-based; and
- Urging local, state, and national support for comprehensive sex education and other health promotion and services for youth by communicating these needs to political officials and by voting for candidates who support these issues.

Vaccination
The Centers for Disease Control and Prevention recommends that all children ages 11 and 12 should be vaccinated against human papillomavirus (HPV) and provides tip sheets for talking to parents about the HPV vaccine (see **Table 3**). HPV can be transmitted through a variety of intimate activities involving contact with genitalia, mucous membranes, or bodily fluids even if the infected person has no signs or symptoms. Early vaccination is optimal but recommended (see Diane R. Blake and Amy B. Middlemans' article, "HPV Vaccine Update," in this issue).

Reproductive health care
The American Academy of Pediatrics (AAP) encourages anticipatory guidance of adolescents in relation to sex beginning at 11 years of age, and parents should begin a dialogue with their child about sexuality at this time if they have not already done so. All adolescents should receive information from their health care providers and parents about where and when to seek reproductive health care and screenings—including locations other than their regular providers, such as free health clinics, county health departments, and the family planning centers. The AAP recently released a clinical report

on sexuality education[11] that reinforces the importance of the pediatrician's role in communicating evidence-based reproductive health and sexuality education and suggests additional resources (included in **Table 3**).

Connectedness with adults who care
Parents are crucial to a child's healthy development, but a supportive, caring relationship with any responsible adult—parent/step-parent, another family member, or friend, teacher, coach, or other—is the most important factor in the development of resilience and avoidance of negative outcomes.[12,13] The ability to adapt to and cope with adversity comes from a network of relationships with trusted adults to create a protective buffer and developmental "scaffolding" that allows children to adapt to adversity and thrive.

Engagement with activities and interests
Overall, involvement with activities and interests promotes positive development. There is some paradoxic evidence when it comes to sports participation, however. Girls' involvement in sports is associated with decreased risky sexual behavior, whereas boys' involvement in sports is associated with increased risky sexual behavior.[14] Sports involvement for girls may increase self-confidence and self-esteem and help them resist traditional gender roles that girls should be sexy, powerless, and compliant. Sports involvement for boys, on the other hand, may be associated with boys subscribing to the traditional role of men. Boys should be encouraged to participate in sports for the benefits, but need to be "inoculated" against stereotypical male gender ideology and behaviors through conversations with parents and other trusted adults about more egalitarian gender roles.

Romantic relationships
Navigating their adolescents' early romantic relationships can be challenging for parents. Adolescents begin experiencing the overpowering emotion of falling in love. This can be problematic because of the lack of emotional regulation and the tendency for relationships at this age to be short term (weeks for younger adolescents, months for middle adolescents, and years for older adolescents and young adults). The emotional intensity involved with falling in love, maintaining a relationship, and breaking up within a short period of time can create a wild ride on an emotional roller coaster. Teens will need guidance as they learn to manage the endings of relationships, a key developmental task.

In addition to emotional risk, adolescent relationships come with other risks. An ongoing intimate relationship with a partner, for example, may put adolescents at increased risk of STIs and unwanted pregnancies, because condom use consistency diminishes with duration of relationships.[15] Teens want to communicate trust and fidelity to their partners, and condom use often diminishes. Parents should watch for and discuss warning signs of current or potential Intimate Partner Violence (IPV) from romantic partners. They should ask questions about whether a partner respects their choices, gives them time and space to spend time with friends, or pressures them to do things they do not want to do (see Futures Without Violence in **Table 3**).

Sexual orientation
A thorough discussion of parent-child communication about sexual orientation is beyond the scope of this article, and sexual orientation, specifically, is addressed in a separate future issue of this journal. Parents are encouraged to approach conversations with their children about sexual orientation with an open mind and to listen more than they speak. "The Gender Unicorn" in **Fig. 1** is a helpful framework to understand

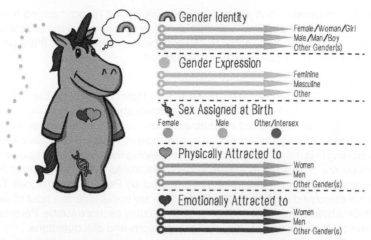

Fig. 1. The gender unicorn. (Design by Landyn Pan and Anna Moore. Trans Student Educational Resources. To learn more, go to: www.transstudent.org/gender.)

the sexual identity spectrum and to establish a common language around gender identity, gender expression, biological sex, and sexual orientation.

Many parents make the mistake of thinking LGBTQIA (lesbian, gay, bisexual, transgender, queer, intersex, asexual) adolescents do not need information on pregnancy prevention because they may not be engaging in sexual behavior with an opposite sex partner, but LGBTQIA adolescents sometimes engage in heterosexual behaviors. There are risks for STIs regardless of the sex of the partner they choose. LGBTQIA teens should receive resources and information about barrier protection as well as ongoing and emergency contraception. Parents of LGBTQIA children and adolescents can seek out supportive groups and resources such as PFLAG (see **Table 3**).

Contraception

Parents will want to review the types of contraception available. Even if parents are encouraging abstinence, teens need to know how contraceptives work and their effectiveness. A well-informed teen is a valuable resource for their peers. **Table 3** suggests resources for medically accurate contraceptive information for providers, parents, and teens (related articles in this issue offer additional guidance).

Media/pornography

Personal portable devices such as smartphones and tablets are increasingly the source of teen's media access, including communication with words, photos, and videos. Images related to sex and alcohol are prevalent, and exposure increases the likelihood of risky sexual attitudes and behaviors.[16,17] Parents should be aware of their child's media consumption, although advances in technology make it increasingly difficult to keep track. "Spot checks" on teen's smartphones and other devices can be conducted, but on some apps (eg, Snapchat) images are only stored temporarily, and it is nearly impossible to know where the user has been. Although it is beyond the scope of this article, a continuing challenge for parents will be to keep up with technological advancements that allow parental monitoring and control of media exposure on personal devices. Parents will also need to have conversations with their teens about interpersonal communication (eg, sexting), how alcohol and other substances affect decision making, portrayals of men and women in the media, and issues related to consent and power in relationships. One recommended resource in **Table 3** is "Ask the Mediatrician," a pediatrician who specializes in the effects of media exposure on children and adolescents. Parents can use this tool for entry points into conversations and send questions to be answered.

Sexual abuse/exploitation

Parents should closely monitor who interacts with their children and the nature of this relationship. Many parent-child conversations about abuse and abduction prevention focus on unknown strangers, but most abusers are known to the children they abuse. Parents should explain abuse to their children from an early age. This explanation should include teaching that only those people who are helping them keep their bodies healthy, clean, or safe are allowed to touch them. Excellent books containing age-appropriate language explaining abuse include those authored by Robie H. Harris (see **Table 3**). Abuse is not the only danger to adolescents; they are vulnerable to a host of exploitive relationships whose symptoms and consequences may be more subtle. Parents should closely monitor their teens' activities and companions and ask questions.

Concrete Tips for Parents for Talking to Adolescents About Sexuality

In light of the best practices for parent-adolescent communication presented, the authors offer concrete tips for parents to help them focus their efforts:

1. Educate yourself first. Ask your provider for resources. Explore them.
2. Consider your own emotions and values and what it is important for you to transmit.
3. Establish a common language for talking about sexuality and create conversational ground rules to foster a nonjudgmental atmosphere.
4. Be clear and candid and admit when you do not know the answer. Working together to find answers may be rewarding. It is always okay to say, "I don't know" or "I need to think about that."
5. Use teachable moments to have conversations related to a variety of topics on a regular basis. Teachable moments include major life events and everyday occurrences, and they can be spontaneous or scripted in advance.
6. Solicit the help of close family and/or friends who may be trusted adults for your child. It is beneficial to have a network of supportive and "askable" adults.
7. Pay attention to what your child is seeing and hearing in the media (television, movies, video games, social media posts, music, and so forth). Monitor social media use and limit Internet access to common family spaces as much as possible. Take advantage of the many teachable moments in the media.
8. Know who is providing sex education to your child and whether the educational content is comprehensive, medically accurate, and evidence based. Be a proponent of comprehensive sex education in your schools and faith-based or community organizations.
9. Identify and communicate about organizations, clinics, and resources in the community that provide access to reproductive health care.
10. Check in regularly about what your child is feeling, seeing, hearing, and experiencing. Listen. Share your own experiences, successes, and mistakes.
11. Understand that what you *do* is the most important message about your values.

SUMMARY

Parents should offer clear, accurate, and developmentally appropriate information about the behaviors expected from their children and how to keep them safe. Parents play a primary role in disseminating sexual information—through words, behaviors, and values they convey. The role of the of the health care provider is to advise parents and direct them to resources so they can approach conversations prepared with knowledge and confidence—to make them "askable" parents. Health care providers have a responsibility to independently and collaboratively address issues with their adolescent patients, respecting standards of confidentiality, in a framework that also includes state-specific child protection mandates. The strategies and resources recommended in this article are intended to help providers guide both parents and adolescents to improve their knowledge of and communication about sexuality matters.

ACKNOWLEDGMENTS

The authors would like to thank Melissa Keyes-DiGioia, CSE, for her insightful comments on an earlier draft of this article.

REFERENCES

1. The National Campaign. Teens say parents most influence their decisions about sex: new survey data of teens and adults released [press release]. Washington, DC: 2012. Available at: https://thenationalcampaign.org/press-release/teens-say-parents-most-influence-their-decisions-about-sex.
2. Karofsky PS, Zeng L, Kosorok MR. Relationship between adolescent-parental communication and initiation of first intercourse by adolescents. J Adolesc Health 2001;28(1):41–5.
3. Miller KS, Levin ML, Whitaker DJ, et al. Patterns of condom use among adolescents: the impact of mother-adolescent communication. Am J Public Health 1998;88(10):1542–4.
4. Weinman ML, Small E, Buzi RS, et al. Risk factors, parental communication, self and peers' beliefs as predictors of condom use among female adolescents attending family planning clinics. Child Adolesc Social Work J 2008;25:157.
5. Ashcraft AM. A qualitative investigation of urban African American mother/daughter communication about relationships and sex [unpublished doctoral dissertation]. Richmond (VA): Virginia Commonwealth University; 2012.
6. Harris RH, Emberley M. It's perfectly normal: changing bodies, growing up, sex, and sexual health. Somerville (MA): Candlewick Press; 2014.
7. Buni C. The case for teaching kids 'vagina,' 'penis,' and 'vulva'. Atlantic 2013.
8. Burger N. Why teaching children anatomically correct words matters. KevinMD.com; 2014. Available at: http://www.kevinmd.com/blog/2014/12/teaching-anatomically-correct-words-matters.html. Accessed July 23, 2014.
9. Trenholm C, Devaney D, Fortson K, et al. Impacts of four title V, section 510 abstinence education programs. Princeton (NJ): Mathematica Policy Research; 2007. Available at: https://aspe.hhs.gov/basic-report/impacts-four-title-v-section-510-abstinence-education-programs. Accessed August 12, 2016.
10. Downs JS. Prescriptive scientific narratives for communicating usable science. Proc Natl Acad Sci U S A 2014;111(Suppl 4):13627–33.
11. Bruener CC, Mattson G, Committee on Adolescence, et al. Sexuality education for children and adolescents. Pediatrics 2016;138(2):e20161348.
12. Resnick MD, Bearman PS, Blum RW, et al. Protecting adolescents from harm: findings from the National Longitudinal Study on Adolescent Health. JAMA 1997;278(10):823–32.

13. Ackard DM, Neumark-Sztainer D, Story M, et al. Parent-child connectedness and behavioral and emotional health among adolescents. Am J Prev Med 2006;30(1): 59–66.
14. Tracy AJ, Erkut S. Gender and race patterns in the pathways from sports partic-ipation to self-esteem. Sociol Perspect 2002;45(4):445–66.
15. Fortenberry JD, Tu W, Harezlak J, et al. Condom use as a function of time in new and established adolescent sexual relationships. Am J Public Health 2002;92(2): 211–3.
16. Bailin A, Milanaik R, Adesman A. Health implications of new age technologies for adolescents: a review of the research. Curr Opin Pediatr 2014;26(5):605–19.
17. Moreno MA, Whitehill JM. Influence of social media on alcohol use in adolescents and young adults. Alcohol Res 2014;36(1):91–100.

Human Papillomavirus Vaccine Update

Diane R. Blake, MD[a],*, Amy B. Middleman, MD, MSEd, MPH[b]

KEYWORDS

- Human papillomavirus • Vaccine • Cervical cancer • Oropharyngeal cancer

KEY POINTS

- Cancers attributable to human papillomavirus (HPV) are on the rise.
- Vaccine against the 7 HPV types that cause 73% of HPV-associated cancers is available, safe, and very effective.
- Vaccine also protects against the 2 HPV types that cause 90% of genital warts.
- The health care provider's recommendation to vaccinate is among the most important determinants of whether a teen receives the HPV vaccine.
- HPV vaccine should be recommended at the 11- or 12-year-old well-child visit and the series should be completed by the 13th birthday.

INTRODUCTION

There are more than 120 different types of human papillomavirus (HPV). Most are responsible for warts found on the skin.[1] Approximately 40 HPV types infect mucosal surfaces and the genital tract,[1] and 13 of these are oncogenic.[2] This article examines the epidemiology and strategies to control the spread of the most common and most serious HPV types for which preventive vaccines are available.

EPIDEMIOLOGY

Approximately 79 million people in the United States are infected with HPV, and 14 million acquire a new infection each year.[3] In 1 study measuring HPV prevalence just before introduction of a quadrivalent HPV vaccine in 2006, 33% of 14- to 19-year-old female patients and 54% of 20-to 24-year-old female patients were infected with genital HPV.[1]

The authors report no commercial or financial conflict of interest.
[a] Department of Pediatrics, University of Massachusetts Medical School, 55 Lake Avenue North, Worcester, MA 01655, USA; [b] Department of Pediatrics, University of Oklahoma Health Sciences Center, 1200 Children's Avenue, Suite 12200, Oklahoma City, OK 73104, USA
* Corresponding author.
E-mail address: diane.blake@umassmed.edu

Pediatr Clin N Am 64 (2017) 321–329
http://dx.doi.org/10.1016/j.pcl.2016.11.003
0031-3955/17/© 2016 Elsevier Inc. All rights reserved.

pediatric.theclinics.com

A systematic review published in 2006 included numerous HPV prevalence studies among men but most studies did not stratify by age. The prevalence in the 8 studies conducted in university or military settings ranged from 10% to 40%.[5] The US cohort of men enrolled into the Human Papillomavirus in Men study had a prevalence of 23% for 15- to 19-year-old, 10% for 25- to 29-year-old, and 37% for 20- to 24-year-old men.[6]

There are differences in race and ethnicity among those who develop HPV-related cancers.[7] For example, Hispanic and black women experience higher rates of cervical cancer than white women, and American Indian or Alaska Native and Asian or Pacific Islander women experience the lowest rates.[8] It is not clear whether these differences are due to access to care and screening issues, innate genetic differences of HPV hosts based on race, or intratypic HPV variants circulating in different community populations.[9] More study is needed.

PATHOPHYSIOLOGY AND NATURAL HISTORY

Most HPV infections have no symptoms and are cleared by the host immune system, usually within 1 to 2 years. However, viral shedding occurs even when no visible lesions are present. Although condoms can prevent transmission of HPV, contact frequently occurs at sites that are not protected by the condom barrier. HPV can also be spread by nonsexual skin-to-skin contact. Therefore, even when partners consistently use condoms, viral transmission can occur.

HPV 6 and 11 are the types that account for approximately 90% of cases of genital warts.[10] Although the HPV types that cause genital warts are nononcogenic, there can still be significant morbidity associated with the development of genital warts, most notably psychological distress as a result of both the appearance and the recurrence of genital warts.

When any of the 13 sexually transmitted oncogenic HPV types persist, precancer and cancer can develop.[11] The time between infection and development of cancer is generally at least 15 years and can be up to 25 years or more.[12] HPV 16 is the type most likely to persist and, therefore, to cause cancer.[11] Immunocompromised individuals, such as those with human immunodeficiency virus (HIV) infection or those who take immunosuppressive medication, are at higher risk for HPV persistence.

BURDEN OF DISEASE

Sexually transmitted HPV-associated cancers include cancers of the cervix, vulva, vagina, penis, oropharynx, anus, and rectum. Oropharyngeal cancers include cancers of the base of the tongue, the pharyngeal tonsils and tonsillar pillars, the anterior surface of the soft palate and uvula, and the lateral and posterior pharyngeal walls.

Analysis of 2008 to 2012 data from the Centers for Disease Control and Prevention's (CDC's) National Program of Cancer Registries and the National Cancer Institute's Surveillance, Epidemiology, and End Results program provides estimates of cancers attributable to HPV.[11] Using information from polymerase chain reaction genotyping studies, the investigators calculated the proportion of HPV-associated cancers that were attributable to an oncogenic HPV type.[11] Of the 30,100 cancers attributable to HPV from 2008 to 2012, 18,700 were in female patients and 11,400 were in male patients (**Table 1**).[11] These data also demonstrated an increase in HPV-related cancers compared with 26,000 diagnoses per year during 2004 to 2008.[13]

The American Cancer Society estimates that 12,990 new cases of invasive cervical cancer will be diagnosed in the United States in 2016 and 4120 women will die from cervical cancer.[14] For vulvar cancer, the estimates are 5950 women will be diagnosed and

Table 1
Annual cancers attributable to human papillomavirus—United States, 2008–2012

Cancer	Average Number of HPV-Associated Cancers		Average Number of Cancers Attributable to HPV	
	Female	Male	Female	Male
Anal	3260	1750	3000	1600
Cervical	11,771	0	10,700	0
Oropharyngeal	3100	12,638	2000	9100
Penile	0	1168	0	700
Vaginal	802	0	600	0
Vulvar	3554	0	2400	0
Total	22,487	15,556	18,700	11,400

Adapted from Viens LJ, Henley SJ, Watson M, et al. Human Papillomavirus-Associated Cancers - United States, 2008-2012. MMWR Morb Mortal Wkly Rep 2016;65(26):661–6.

1110 women will die.[15] For anal cancer, the estimates are 8080 new cases and 1080 deaths.[16] The CDC estimates that 9000 new cases of oropharyngeal cancer due to HPV occur each year, with 4 times as many of these cancers occurring in men than in women.[17] The 5-year survival rate for oropharyngeal cancer is 85% to 90%.[18]

Data from the early 2000s suggest that the annual incidence of anogenital warts is approximately 225 per 100,000, and equally distributed between men and women.[19] It is estimated that 1.2 per 1000 female patients and 1.1 per 1000 male patients have acquired genital warts,[20] with the peak incidence in women occurring between the ages of 20 to 24 years and the peak incidence in men occurring between 25 to 29 years.[21]

AVAILABLE VACCINES FOR PREVENTION

Before 2017, there were 3 types of vaccine available to protect against HPV in the United States: bivalent (2vHPV), quadrivalent (4vHPV), and 9-valent (9vHPV) (**Table 2**). All 3 vaccines protect against HPV types 16 and 18, which cause 63% of HPV-associated cancers in the United States. Although 2vHPV and 4vHPV vaccines

Table 2
Advisory Committee on Immunization Practices updated recommendations March, 2015

	Bivalent (Cervix)	Quadrivalent (Gardasil)	9-Valent (Gardasil 9)
Manufacturer	GlaxoSmithKline	Merck	Merck
HPV types	16, 18	6, 11, 16, 18	6, 11, 16, 18, 31, 33, 45, 52, 58
Recommended age[a]	Female patients 11–26 y	Female patients 11–26 y Male patients 11–21 y[b]	Female patients 11–26 y Male patients 11–21 y[b]

[a] HPV vaccine may be given as young as age 9 years.
[b] Immunization through age 26 years is recommended for men who have sex with men; men who are immunocompromised, including infection with HIV; and all men desiring protection against HPV.

Adapted from Petrovsky E, Bocchini JA Jr, Hariri S, et al. Use of 9-valent human papillomavirus (HPV) vaccine: updated HPV vaccination recommendations of the advisory committee on immunization practices. MMWR Morb Mortal Wkly Rep 2015;64:300–4.

are still available outside of the United States, currently only the 9-valent product is used in the Unites States.[22] The 4vHPV and 9vHPV vaccines protect against HPV types 6 and 11, which cause 90% of genital warts. The 9-valent vaccine, licensed in 2015, includes protection against 5 additional oncogenic HPV types that cause an additional 10% of HPV-associated cancers in the United States.[11]

The Advisory Committee on Immunization Practices (ACIP) recommends that adolescents begin the HPV vaccination series at age 11 to 12 years (see **Table 2**) and complete the series by their 13th birthday. The vaccine is most effective when administered before initiation of sexual activity because the vaccines are preventive only and do not treat or cure HPV infection that has already occurred nor dysplasia or cancer that has developed in response to HPV infection.[12] The vaccine may be administered as early as 9 years of age. The vaccination series should be administered routinely to young men through the age of 21 years who have not previously received the vaccine. Men having sex with men, men who are immunocompromised, and all men desiring protection from HPV infection should receive the vaccination series through the age of 26 years. All young women through age 26 years who have not previously been vaccinated should receive the vaccination series.[23] For those who initiate the series at age 9 through 14 years of age, a 2-dose series is administered with the second dose 6 to 12 months after the first dose; for those 15 years of age or older at the time of the first dose, a 3-dose series is recommended. When giving the 3-dose series, the second dose should be given 2 months following the first dose, with a minimum interval of 4 weeks between doses 1 and 2. The third dose should be given at least 24 weeks after the first dose and at least 12 weeks after the second dose (**Table 3**).[23,24]

IMMUNOGENICITY

Younger individuals have more robust antibody responses to the HPV vaccine, with antibody response decreasing with older age at vaccination. Older adolescents and young adults still have a greater than 99% seroconversion to antibody types contained in the vaccines; however, the magnitude of antibody response is higher among 9- to 15-year-old compared with 16- to 26-year-old patients.[23]

Studies to date demonstrate long-term immune memory following the standard 3-dose series with no evidence of waning immunity.[12] Although initial immune response is similar between a 3-dose schedule among female patients 16 to 26 years of age and 2 doses given at least 6 months apart for younger girls age 9 to 15 years of age, long-term efficacy data are not yet available from 2-dose trials.[12]

EFFICACY AND SAFETY

Cervical cancer develops over many years. Therefore, it is not a feasible endpoint for vaccine efficacy studies. Clinical trials on the quadrivalent vaccine instead used prevention of cervical intraepithelial neoplasia (CIN)-2 as the primary endpoint. Not all CIN2 lesions

Table 3
HPV dosing and timing of 9-valent vaccine[24]

Age at 1st Dose	Regimen	Minimum Time bw 1st & 2nd Dose	Minimum Time bw 2nd and 3rd Dose	Minimum Time bw 1st and 3rd Dose
9–14 y	2-dose	24 wk	NA	NA
15–26 y	3-dose	4 wk	12 wk	24 wk

Advisory Committee on Immunization Practices (ACIP) Meeting 10/20/16

will develop into cervical cancer but the risk is high enough that this degree of dysplasia requires treatment. On the other hand, milder lesions, such as CIN1 and atypical squamous cells of undetermined significance, often resolve spontaneously and can be monitored. In the quadrivalent vaccine trials, nearly 100% of those in the vaccine groups were protected against CIN2 caused by HPV 16 and 18. Likewise, nearly all of those in the vaccine group were protected against genital warts due to HPV 6 and 11 and from vulvar, vaginal, and anal dysplasia due to HPV types in the vaccine.[12]

Prevalence studies conducted in the United States through 2010 demonstrated a 50% decrease in prevalence of vaccine type HPV among these women aged 14 to 24 years. A more recent study found a 40% reduction in vaccine type HPV prevalence among women ages 20 to 29 years who were screened in 2012 to 2013 compared with those screened in 2007.[25] A recent study found that the prevalence of vaccine type HPV decreased by nearly two-thirds in girls and women since the introduction of the quadrivalent vaccine.[26]

Clinical trials of the 9vHPV vaccine have demonstrated greater than 96% efficacy against new persistent cervical infections and CIN2 due to the additional 5 HPV types in this vaccine.[23] Although not currently recommended by ACIP, it is safe to revaccinate those who have received 4vHPV vaccine with a 3-dose series.[27]

Postlicensure monitoring of quadrivalent vaccine safety has not identified serious safety concerns and results are consistent with prelicensing trial data.[10,28] The most common side effects are pain and swelling at the injection site, dizziness, syncope, nausea, and headache.[10]

VACCINE UPTAKE

The CDC uses the annual National Immunization Survey–Teen (NIS-Teen) to monitor vaccine coverage. Data from the most recent survey in 2015 showed that 49.8% of male and 62.8% of female adolescents between the age of 13 and 17 years had received at least one dose of the HPV series.[29] This is in stark contrast to 86.4% and 81.3% of youth in the same age group having received at least one dose of Tdap and meningococcal conjugate vaccine, respectively (**Table 4**).[29] Furthermore, only 28.1% of boys and 41.9% of girls received all three HPV doses.[29]

TABLE 4 National Immunization Survey: teen coverage results 2008–2015								
Vaccine	2008	2009	2010	2011	2012	2013	2014	2015
Tdap after 10 y of age, %	40.8	55.6	68.7	78.2	84.6	86.0	87.6	86.4
≥3 doses HepB, %	87.9	89.9	91.6	92.3	92.8	93.2	91.4	91.1
≥2 doses MMR, %	89.3	89.1	90.5	91.1	91.4	91.8	90.7	90.7
≥2 doses of Varicella, %	34.1	48.6	58.1	68.3	74.9	78.5	81.0	83.1
≥1 MCV4, %	41.8	53.6	62.7	70.5	74.0	77.8	79.3	81.3
HPV								
Females								
≥1 dose, %	37.2	44.3	48.7	53.0	53.8	57.3	60.0	62.8
≥3 doses, %	17.9	26.7	32.0	34.8	33.4	37.6	39.7	41.9
Males								
≥1 dose, %	—	—	1.4	8.3	20.8	34.6	41.7	49.8
≥3 doses, %	—	—	—	1.3	6.8	13.9	21.6	28.1

Data from Reagan-Steiner S, Yankey D, Jeyarajah J, et al. National, regional, state, and selected local area vaccination coverage among adolescents aged 13–17 years - United States, 2015. MMWR Morb Mortal Wkly Rep 2016;65:850–8.

NIS-Teen data from 2013 demonstrated that, for parents of both boys and girls, not receiving a recommendation to vaccinate and not knowing enough about the HPV vaccine were among the top 5 reasons for not having their child vaccinated against HPV.[28] Partly in response to these data, a study published in 2015 investigated physician communication about HPV vaccine.[30] A national sample of 776 pediatricians and family physicians completed online surveys about strength of endorsement, timeliness, consistency, and urgency of recommendations to vaccinate. A sizable minority recommended beginning vaccine series after the 13th birthday for boys (39%) and girls (26%), not during the current visit (49%), and with lower strength of endorsement (27%).[30] A majority reported using a risk-based approach (59%) to determine to whom to recommend vaccine.[30] It is concerning that so many physicians in the sample discussed the vaccine in a way that was likely to discourage parents from immunizing their child.

It is not clear why providers often discuss the HPV vaccine in a different way to parents and patients. One recent study reveals that providers have a belief that parents do not think that the HPV vaccine is as important to their child's health as other childhood vaccines.[31] In this study, researchers asked parents how important they thought various vaccines were to their child's health and then asked providers to predict how parents responded. Providers inaccurately and grossly underestimated the importance parents place on adolescent vaccines in general and HPV vaccine in particular (**Fig. 1**).[31]

Much work is being done to understand how to most effectively approach parents and patients regarding the HPV vaccine. The CDC has developed talking points to help providers address any parental concerns (http://www.cdc.gov/cancer/knowledge/provider-education/hpv/index.htm). It is critical that providers create a message that emphasizes a strong recommendation.[32]

Some states and local areas have much better HPV vaccine uptake than the country as a whole. Those that have been successful in improving vaccine coverage have used several strategies, including cancer prevention and immunization stakeholders working together because many states with the highest cervical cancer rates have the poorest HPV vaccination uptake rates, comprehensive public communication campaigns, and using all opportunities to educate clinicians and parents about the importance of on-time HPV vaccination.[33]

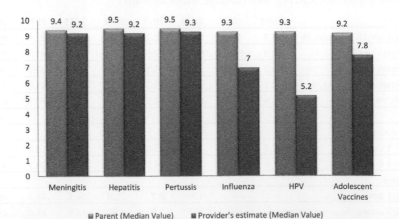

Fig. 1. Clinicians underestimate the value parents place on HPV vaccine. (*From* Centers for Disease Control. You are the key to HPV cancer prevention. Available at: https://www.cdc.gov/vaccines/ed/hpv/index.html. Accessed December 2, 2016.)

SUMMARY

Rates of cancers attributable to HPV are rising. The morbidity and mortality of these cancers place an unnecessary burden of disease on the US population and on the US health care budget. A safe and extremely effective vaccine is available to prevent many of these cancers.

Studies have shown that the health care provider's recommendation to immunize is the most important factor in the parent's decision. Parents of all adolescent boys and girls should receive a strong and unequivocal recommendation to vaccinate their child against HPV at the 11- or 12-year-old well-child visit. This recommendation should be consistent with the recommendation to receive the Tdap and MCV4 vaccines. Ideally, adolescents will complete their HPV vaccine series by the 13th birthday. This will lead to greater immune response and protect most adolescents before they are exposed to sexually transmitted HPV.

REFERENCES

1. Markowitz L, Unger E. Human papillomaviruses. The pink book: epidemiology and prevention of vaccine-preventable diseases. Atlanta (GA): Centers for Disease Control and Prevention; 2015. p. 1–12.
2. Centers for Disease Control and Prevention. Sexually transmitted diseases treatment guidelines, 2015. MMWR Recomm Rep 2015;64(No. RR-3):1–137.
3. Centers for Disease Control and Prevention. Human Papillomavirus (HPV). 2016. Available at: http://www.cdc.gov/std/hpv/stdfact-hpv.htm. Accessed August 3, 2016.
4. Hariri S, Unger ER, Sternberg M, et al. Prevalence of genital human papillomavirus among females in the United States, the National Health and nutrition examination survey, 2003-2006. J Infect Dis 2011;204(4):566–73.
5. Dunne EF, Nielson CM, Stone KM, et al. Prevalence of HPV infection among men: a systematic review of the literature. J Infect Dis 2006;194:1044–57.
6. Giuliano AR, Lazcano-Ponce E, Villa LL, et al. The human papillomavirus infection in men study: human papillomavirus prevalence and type distribution among men residing in Brazil, Mexico, and the United States. Cancer Epidemiol Biomarkers Prev 2008;17(8):2036–43.
7. Centers for Disease Control and Prevention. HPV-Associated Cancers Rates by Race and Ethnicity. 2016. Available at: http://www.cdc.gov/cancer/hpv/statistics/race.htm. Accessed August 3, 2016.
8. Centers for Disease Control and Prevention. Cervical Cancer Rates by Race and Ethnicity. 2016. Available at: http://www.cdc.gov/cancer/cervical/statistics/race.htm. Accessed August 3, 2016.
9. Schabath MB, Villa LL, Lin H-Y, et al. Racial differences in the incidence and clearance of human papilloma virus (HPV): The HPV in men (HIM) study. Cancer Epidemiol Biomarkers Prev 2013;22(10):1762–70.
10. Stokley S, Curtis CR, Jeyarajah J, et al. Human papillomavirus vaccination coverage among adolescent girls, 2007–2012, and postlicensure vaccine safety monitoring, 2006–2013 — United States. MMWR Morb Mortal Wkly Rep 2013;62(29):591–5.
11. Viens LJ, Henley SJ, Watson M, et al. Human papillomavirus-associated cancers - United States, 2008-2012. MMWR Morb Mortal Wkly Rep 2016;65(26):661–6.
12. Lowy DR. HPV vaccination to prevent cervical cancer and other HPV-associated disease: from basic science to effective interventions. J Clin Invest 2016;126(1):5–11.

13. Wu X, Watson M, Wilson R, et al. Human papillomavirus-associated cancers - United States, 2004-2008. MMWR Morb Mortal Wkly Rep 2012;61(15):258–61.

14. American Cancer Society. What are the key statistics about cervical cancer? 2016. Available at: http://www.cancer.org/cancer/cervicalcancer/detailedguide/cervical-cancer-key-statistics. Accessed June 23, 2016.

15. American Cancer Society. What are the key statistics about vulvar cancer? 2016. Available at: http://www.cancer.org/cancer/vulvarcancer/detailedguide/vulvar-cancer-key-statistics. Accessed June 23, 2016.

16. American Cancer Society. What are the key statistics about anal cancer? 2016. Available at: http://www.cancer.org/cancer/analcancer/detailedguide/anal-cancer-what-is-key-statistics. Accessed July 13, 2016.

17. Centers for Disease Control and Prevention. HPV and Oropharyngeal Cancer - Fact Sheet. 2016. http://www.cdc.gov/std/hpv/stdfact-hpvandoropharyngealcancer.htm. Accessed August 6, 2016.

18. Mount Sinai Hospital. Human HPV and Throat/Oral Cancer Frequently Asked Questions. 2016. Available at: http://www.mountsinai.org/patient-care/service-areas/ent/areas-of-care/head-and-neck-cancer/oral-cancer/hpv/hpv-faq. Accessed August 6, 2016.

19. Patel H, Wagner M, Singhal P, et al. Systematic review of incidence and prevalence of genital warts. BMC Infect Dis 2013;13:39.

20. Markowitz LE, Dunne EF, Saraiya M, et al. Human papillomavirus vaccination: recommendations of the Advisory Committee on Immunization Practices (ACIP). MMWR Recomm Rep 2014;63(RR05):1–30.

21. Flagg EW, Schwartz R, Weinstock H. Prevalence of anogenital warts among participants in private health plans in the United States, 2003–2010: potential impact of human papillomavirus vaccination. Am J Public Health 2013;103(8):1428–35.

22. Markowitz LE. HPV Vaccine Availability, United States. Paper presented at: Presentation at ACIP, Centers for Disease Control and Prevention. Atlanta, GA, June 23, 2016.

23. Petrosky E, Bocchini JA, Chesson H, et al. Use of 9-valent human papilloma virus (HPV) vaccine: updated HPV vaccination recommendations of the Advisory Committee on Immunization Practices. MMWR Morb Mortal Wkly Rep 2015;64:300–4.

24. Jenco M. ACIP updates recommendations on HPV, HepB, MenB vaccines. AAP News. October 20, 2016.

25. Dunne EF, Naleway A, Smith N, et al. Reduction in human papillomavirus vaccine type prevalence among young women screened for cervical cancer in an integrated US healthcare delivery system in 2007 and 2012-2013. J Infect Dis 2015;212:1970–5.

26. Markowitz LE, Liu G, Hariri S, et al. Prevalence of HPV after introduction of the vaccination program in the United States. Pediatrics 2016;137(3):1–11.

27. Centers for Disease Control and Prevention. Supplemental information and guidance for vaccination providers regarding use of 9-valent HPV vaccine. Atlanta (GA): CDC; 2015. Available at: https://www.cdc.gov/hpv/downloads/9vhpv-guidance.pdf. Accessed December 2, 2016.

28. Stokley S, Jeyarajah J, Yankey D, et al. Human papillomavirus vaccination coverage among adolescents, 2007-2013, postlicensure vaccine safety monitoring, 2006-2014-United States. MMWR Morb Mortal Wkly Rep 2014;63(29):620–4.

29. Reagan-Steiner S, Yankey D, Jeyarajah J, et al. National, regional, state, and selected local area vaccination coverage among adolescents aged 13-17 years - United States, 2015. MMWR Morb Mortal Wkly Rep 2016;65(33):850–8.

30. Gilkey MB, Malo TL, Shah PD, et al. Quality of physician communication about human papillomavirus vaccine: findings from a national survey. Cancer Epidemiol Biomarkers Prev 2015;24(11):1673–9.
31. Healey CM, Montesinos DP, Middleman AB. Parent and provider perspectives on immunization: are providers overestimating parental concerns? Vaccine 2014; 32(5):579–84.
32. Gilkey MB, Calo WA, Moss JL, et al. Provider communication and HPV vaccination: the impact of recommendation quality. Vaccine 2016;34(9):1187–92.
33. Centers for Disease Control and Prevention. For Parents: Vaccines for Your Children - Teen Vaccination Coverage. 2015. Available at: http://www.cdc.gov/vaccines/parents/vacc-coverage-teens.html. Accessed July 13, 2016.

The Treatment of Dysmenorrhea

Sheryl A. Ryan, MD

KEYWORDS

- Adolescent • Menstrual problems • Dysmenorrhea • Menorrhagia
- Excessive uterine bleeding

KEY POINTS

- The time between menarche and the establishment of ovulatory menstrual cycles is variable but may take as long as 2 to 4 years.
- Primary dysmenorrhea is a clinical diagnosis rarely requiring extensive diagnostic tests and is generally responsive to graded management using nonsteroidal anti-inflammatory drugs (NSAIDs) and combined oral contraceptives.
- Excessive uterine bleeding can be seen as a consequence of physiologic anovulation from an immature hypothalamic-pituitary-gonadal axis but when it occurs soon after menarche bleeding diathesis must be considered.
- When evaluating dysmenorrhea, the history and physical examination provide important clues to etiologic factors and guide the diagnostic evaluations that may be needed.
- Evidence is available to support the use of both NSAIDs and hormonal treatments for the management of primary dysmenorrhea.

INTRODUCTION

Menstrual disorders and abnormal uterine bleeding are common concerns that bring young women to the physician's office. Complaints include menses that are too painful (dysmenorrhea), are absent or occur irregularly (amenorrhea or oligoamenorrhea), or are prolonged and heavy (menorrhagia, or excessive uterine bleeding). In providing optimal reproductive care to these adolescents, the medical provider must be able to distinguish normal developmental patterns or symptoms requiring education and reassurance from pathologic conditions requiring prompt assessment and treatment. This article is a discussion of the normal menstrual patterns seen in adolescent females with an evaluation and management approach to primary and secondary dysmenorrhea.

The author declares that she has no financial conflicts of interest related the preparation or content of this article.
Section of Adolescent Medicine, Department of Pediatrics, Yale University School of Medicine, PO Box 208064, 330 Cedar Street, New Haven, CT 06520, USA
E-mail address: Sheryl.ryan@yale.edu

NORMAL MENSTRUAL PATTERNS IN ADOLESCENTS

Normal menstrual cycles require the maturation of the complex feedback system of the hypothalamic-pituitary-gonadal (H-P-G) axis. The mature system involves orderly and sequential release from the pituitary of luteinizing hormone (LH) and follicle-stimulating hormone (FSH), in response to gonadotropin-releasing hormone from the hypothalamus. This results in the growth and maturation of follicles in the ovary, oocyte maturation, and estrogen and progesterone secretion. In the initial follicular phase of a normal menstrual cycle, increasing levels of FSH stimulate the maturation of an ovarian follicle as well as the secretion of estrogen. Estrogen, in turn, stimulates endometrial proliferation. In an ovulatory midcycle, the rising level of estrogen switches from a negative feedback mechanism on both LH and FSH to a positive mechanism. The resulting surge of LH precipitates the release of an oocyte from a mature follicle. The second half of the menstrual cycle, the luteal phase, is character-ized primarily by secretion of progesterone as well as estrogen by the corpus luteum formed by the residual follicle. This results in falling levels of FSH and LH, and some additional growth but also stabilization of the thickened endometrium. In the absence of pregnancy and implantation, after about 10 to 14 days, the corpus luteum involutes, and estrogen and progesterone levels decline, resulting in endometrial shedding, or menstruation. In most adult women, this cycle averages 28 days but can vary from 24 to 35 days and typically lasts 4 to 6 days.

Ovulatory menstrual cycles occur at varying rates following menarche. Within 2 years of menarche, 18% to 45% of female patients will have established regular ovulatory cycles. This increases to 45% to 70% by 2 to 4 years following menarche and to 80% by 5 years.[1] Dysmenorrhea generally occurs during ovulatory cycles, explaining why most dysmenorrhea in adolescents usually has onset 6 to 12 months following menarche. Dysmenorrhea can occur less frequently, however, even with anovulatory cycles. Studies have shown that girls who experience menarche earlier generally establish ovulatory cycles within a shorter time than those girls whose menarche occurs later in age.[2]

Before the establishment of ovulatory cycles, follicular development that does not result in ovulation still can produce levels of estrogen that stimulate endometrial pro-liferation. Eventually the negative feedback effect of this level of estrogen will reduce gonadotropins, resulting in falling levels of estrogen and a withdrawal bleed. In this sit-uation, the lack of progesterone to stabilize the endometrium can result in cycles that are prolonged and excessive. This anovulatory excessive bleeding is physiologic and will usually resolve with maturation of the H-P-G axis and the establishment of ovula-tory cycles.

Typical parameters for uterine bleeding considered to be excessive include a dura-tion lasting more than 7 days, reports of perceived flow that is heavier than normal (quantified as more than 80 mL/cycle), cycles occurring less than every 24 days or more than 35 days, and any bleeding between normal cycles.[3,4]

Dysmenorrhea, or painful menses, is a commonly experienced symptom in women of reproductive age. When severe enough, it can result in restrictions in normal func-tioning, such as attending school or work. There are 2 commonly defined categories of dysmenorrhea: primary and secondary. Primary dysmenorrhea refers to pain during menses in the absence of any specific pathologic state and is characterized by recur-rent, crampy, bilateral lower abdominal pain. Secondary dysmenorrhea refers to pain during menses that can be explained by an organic pathologic condition or any disor-der that is determined to be responsible for the reported symptoms of pain with menstruation.

EPIDEMIOLOGY

Dysmenorrhea is considered the most common symptom of all menstrual complaints, especially during middle and later adolescence. Prevalence rates range from 67% to 90% in young women between the ages of 17 and 24 years.[5] A systematic review conducted by the World Health Organization (WHO) in 2006 found the prevalence of menstrual pain in reproductive-aged women to be between 17% and 81%.[6] This review, however, found that severe dysmenorrhea was reported in only 12% to 14% of community-based samples of women in the United Kingdom. Despite that many of these studies use different populations and criteria for assessing the severity of symptoms, these ranges are similar to many previous studies and confirm the high prevalence of this symptom.

Risk factors for dysmenorrhea include younger age (<30 years), early age of menarche (<12 years), nulliparity, and low body mass index (<20).[7,8] The higher rates of dysmenorrhea among women with a strong family history of dysmenorrhea have been postulated to be the result not only of genetic factors but also possibly through conditioned behavior learned from one's mother or sisters or similar family lifestyles.[9] Family history of dysmenorrhea, onset of menarche before age 12 years, and reports of irregular or heavy menstrual flow or longer duration of menstrual bleeding episodes have also been reported as increased risk factors for dysmenorrhea.[9] A limited number of studies also suggest a positive association between depression and/or somatization and dysmenorrhea.[8] The mechanism for this is poorly understood but it is postulated that mental distress can disrupt several neuroendocrine responses, such as impairment of follicular development, progesterone synthesis, prostaglandin activity, and adrenaline and cortisol release.[10] A recent meta-analysis from Britain did not find significant differences in reports of dysmenorrhea by race or ethnicity, and no consistent data have been reported for obesity, alcohol or tobacco use, education, or marital status as risk factors.[7]

PATHOPHYSIOLOGY

Primary dysmenorrhea results from excessive production of prostaglandins at the time of ovulatory menses.[11,12] In the second half of an ovulatory cycle, the withdrawal of progesterone from the normally involuting corpus luteum causes the release of phospholipids, in particular omega-6 fatty acids, which, in turn, are initially converted to arachidonic acid, and then to prostaglandins.[13] This production of prostaglandin results in increased intrauterine pressure and abnormal uterine contractions. In addition, vasoconstriction of uterine vessels results in decreased blood flow, ischemia of the uterine muscles, and increased sensitivity of pain receptors, all of which cause pelvic pain.[14] Endometrial blood flow has been shown to decrease during these uterine contractions, suggesting that the resulting ischemia is responsible for the pain.[15] Prostaglandins are also converted to leukotrienes that, along with the prostaglandin F2-alpha, are also responsible for the systemic symptoms, such as nausea, vomiting, headache, and dizziness, that may accompany menstrual cramps. The requirement for ovulatory cycles to be present for primary dysmenorrhea to occur in part explains why most adolescents will not develop dysmenorrhea with initial menarche but may have pain after they have established more regular menses several months after menarche.

PATIENT EVALUATION OVERVIEW

Primary dysmenorrhea generally coincides with onset of ovulatory cycles. Localized symptoms include lower abdominal pain or pelvic pain, with or without radiation to the lower back or thighs. The pain generally begins with the onset of the menstrual period and can last anywhere from 8 to 72 hours in duration. Additionally, common systemic symptoms are headache (59%), dizziness (28%), fatigue (67%), nausea (55%) or vomiting (24%), and back pain (56%).[13]

As with any physical complaint referable to the genitourinary system in an adolescent, the evaluation of menstrual pain must include a comprehensive history as well as a physical examination with components determined by the history. This is important to rule out any possible pathologic causes for the menstrual pain, as well as to determine the best approach for management. In the sexually active female, it is essential to include a comprehensive sexual history, which is best done separately from the parents, to assure confidentiality of the information obtained.

CLINICAL ASSESSMENT
History

The history should include questions in the following areas:

- Menstrual history
- Specific therapies attempted and their success
- Family history of dysmenorrhea
- Sexual history
- Review of systems (ROS) focusing on systemic, gastrointestinal (GI), genitourinary (GU), musculoskeletal, and psychosocial areas

Box 1 provides specifics areas in the history that need to be considered.

Physical Examination

A general physical examination should be done when the history and ROS point to a possible systemic or non-GU cause for the pain.

A pelvic examination is essential in adolescents who are sexually active, and who report severe pain or limitation of activity, or who have not responded to first and second line treatments for dysmenorrhea.

In a nonsexually active adolescent, with a history that indicates no systemic disease, but is typical for primary dysmenorrhea, a pelvic examination as part of the initial evaluation may not be necessary. In all other adolescents a complete pelvic examination is indicated; with primary dysmenorrhea the pelvic examination is normal. The external genital examination is important for determining sexual maturity rating, the presence of a normal perineal opening, or signs of trauma. The speculum examination is important in determining whether any anatomic conditions are involved, such as outflow obstruction, or the presence of vaginal or cervical discharge, suggestive of infection. The bimanual examination can provide clues as to whether the uterus is nontender, mobile, of normal size, and texture, and whether there are any masses, such as fibroids. The adnexa and uterosacral ligaments should be palpated for tenderness, masses, and nodularity consistent with endometriomas. In a nonsexually active female, a recto-abdominal examination can provide similar information.

DIFFERENTIAL DIAGNOSIS

When obtaining the history from an adolescent, and completing the physical and pelvic examination, several causes need to be considered, before it can be concluded that primary dysmenorrhea is the cause for the menstrual pain, even though almost 90% of dysmenorrhea in an adolescent is primary. Table 1 lists causes for gynecologic-associated menstrual pain, both primary and secondary, as well as their clinical

---

Box 1
Components of the medical history: dysmenorrhea

Menstrual history

- Age at menarche
- History and characteristic of menstrual cycles
  - Interval between periods
  - Typical duration of menses
  - Nature of flow
  - Dates of most recent menses: last menstrual period (LMP) and previous last menstrual period
    - The pediatrician may need to educate the teen that the LMP begins on the first day of menses, and not on the last day.
  - Pattern of menses (irregular vs regular)
  - History of when menstrual pain developed following menarche
  - Characteristics of menstrual pain (location, nature, timing related to onset of menses, duration, associated systemic symptoms, and severity)
  - Extent of functional impairment of activities, such as school, work, typical activities
  - Whether lower abdominal cramping is present at other times in the menstrual cycle
  - Acuity or chronicity of reported pain
- Any therapies that have been used in the past and the response to these
  - Including medications (types, specific doses and duration of treatment), conservative measures (heating pads, exercise) and complementary alternative treatments, such as supplement, herbal remedies, vitamins.
- Family history of dysmenorrhea

Sexual history

- History of sexual activity
- Age of coitarche
- Numbers of prior sexual partners
- History of any sexually transmitted infections
- Presence of dyspareunia
- Contraceptive use, presently and in the past.

ROS

- Probe for any systemic symptoms or symptoms that may indicate a pathologic cause of menstrual pain.
  - Generalized systemic symptoms, such as fatigue, dizziness, or premenstrual physical or emotional symptoms
  - GI symptoms, such as vomiting, diarrhea, pain on defecation, (these may be present in primary dysmenorrhea or may be seen in endometriosis)
  - GU symptoms
  - Musculoskeletal symptoms, particularly in the hip and pelvic are (to rule out possible trauma or tumor as cause of pain)
  - Psychosocial history (to evaluate for substance abuse, especially tobacco smoking, and stress, anxiety, or history of sexual abuse).

---

features, and the diagnostic evaluations that may be indicated. Of note, is that when menarche is associated with significant pain, one needs to suspect an outflow obstruction.[16,17] A noncommunicating uterine horn is an obstructive müllerian anomaly that is seen with menstrual flow. Obstructive anomalies such as imperforate hymen, transverse vaginal septum, or vaginal agenesis should be considered with the onset of acute

Table 1
Differential diagnosis of dysmenorrhea, clinical features, and suggested diagnostic evaluation

Condition	Clinical Features	Evaluation
Primary dysmenorrhea	Recurrent, crampy, suprapubic pain occurring at start of menses, lasting 2–3 d, often accompanied by systemic symptoms	Diagnosis is clinical Should rule out pregnancy
Endometriosis	Cyclic (can be noncyclic) pain with menses Associated with deep dyspareunia, dysuria, dyschezia, and fertility problems Decreased mobility of uterus on examination, adnexal masses, and uterosacral nodularity	Transvaginal and pelvic ultrasound highly accurate for bowel and ovarian endometriomas MRI may be indicated for deep infiltrating endometriomas Laparoscopy with biopsy is preferred diagnostic test
Pelvic inflammatory disease	Lower abdominal pain in sexually active female Abnormal findings on examination: cervical motion tenderness, uterine and adnexal tenderness, cervical or vaginal mucopurulent discharge May have systemic signs, temperature >38.3°C	Cervical infection with *Chlamydia trachomatis* or *Neisseria gonorrhoeae* confirmatory May have elevated erythrocyte sedimentation rate or C-reactive protein Transvaginal ultrasound usually not indicated
Adenomyosis	Usually associated with menorrhagia and intermenstrual bleeding Enlarged, tender, boggy uterus on examination	Transvaginal ultrasound or MRI will detect endometrial tissue within the endometrium
Leiomyomata	Cyclic pelvic pain, usually with menorrhagia Occasional dyspareunia	Transvaginal ultrasound will detect fibroids
Ectopic pregnancy	History of preceding amenorrhea, abnormal uterine bleeding Acute, severe lower abdominal pain Cramping on affected side May present with blood loss, hypovolemia	Positive urine human chorionic gonadotropin pregnancy test Pelvic or transvaginal ultrasound will show lack of intrauterine gestational sac or extrauterine gestational sac
Interstitial cystitis	Suprapubic pain, usually noncyclic, with urinary symptoms (frequency, urgency) Radiation of pain to groin and rectum Normal pelvic examination	Urinalysis Cystoscopy with biopsy, showing bladder wall mucosal irritation
Chronic pelvic pain	History of noncyclic pain for at least 6 mo May radiate toward vagina or rectum May be worsened by anxiety; often associated with dyspareunia, pain on defecation Burning pain unilaterally on rectal examination may suggest pudendal nerve entrapment	Pelvic MRI along pudendal nerve to assess nerve and surrounding structures With negative workup, diagnosis may be based on clinical history

Adapted from Osayande A, Mehulic S. Diagnosis and initial management of dysmenorrhea. Am Fam Physician 2014;89:341–6.

pelvic pain, in the absence of menses in a teen whose Sexual Maturity Rating is advanced enough for menarche to have occurred. In these situations, pelvic or transvaginal ultrasound can identify whether the pelvic and uterine anatomy is normal or associated with these structural anomalies. In addition, several nongynecologic conditions should be considered. These include GI causes (irritable bowel syndrome, inflammatory bowel disease, chronic constipation, and lactose intolerance), GU causes (cystitis, renal calculi), and psychogenic causes (trauma, history of sexual abuse).

DIAGNOSTIC EVALUATION

As listed in **Table 1**, with a history consistent with primary dysmenorrhea and a normal physical and/or pelvic examination (if indicated), no further laboratory or diagnostic tests are indicated. If an underlying cause for the menstrual pain is suspected, several laboratory tests or diagnostic studies may be indicated and judiciously done.

TREATMENT

The overall goal of treatment of dysmenorrhea is the reduction of reported pain and associated systemic symptoms, as well as improved function, such as fewer days lost from work, school, or extracurricular activities.

Pharmacologic Treatment Options

Primary dysmenorrhea

The goal of pharmacologic therapies is to reduce the production of prostaglandins and leukotrienes responsible for the menstrual pain and associated systemic effects. First-line therapies are thus aimed at the reduction of prostaglandins and leukotrienes, through the use of nonsteroidal anti-inflammatory drugs (NSAIDs) and/or hormonal contraceptives.

Nonsteroidal anti-inflammatory drugs The support for the efficacy of NSAIDs lies in their ability to inhibit the enzymes of the cyclooxygenase (COX)-1 and COX-2 pathways that metabolize the fatty acid arachidonic acid to prostaglandin. Both of the classes of NSAIDs, those that are nonspecific and inhibit both COX-1 and COX-2 (ibuprofen, naproxen, diclofenac potassium, and meclofenamate) and those that are specific for COX-2 only (celecoxib, rofecoxib, and valdecoxib), are effective in the treatment of dysmenorrhea. However, because of evidence linking COX-2 inhibitors to cardiac complications, they are no longer recommended for the treatment of dysmenorrhea.[13] The action of NSAIDs on COX-1 inhibition is also responsible for the side effects of GI upset and renal failure; these can be minimized with short-term use.

A 2010 Cochrane review of 73 randomized controlled trials reported strong evidence to support the use of NSAIDs as the first-line treatment of primary dysmenorrhea and up to 80% of patients will respond to them.[18] No NSAID has been proven more effective than any other. Thus, the choice of which preparation to use should be based on patient preference, and the tolerability and efficacy for each individual patient. It is recommended that all NSAIDs should be taken, if possible, 1 to 2 days before the start of the menses, preferably with a loading dose and continued regularly for the first 2 to 3 days of menstrual bleeding or for the duration of the cramping. Recommended doses of specific NSAIDs are listed in **Table 2**.

Hormonal Agents

The data supporting the efficacy of hormonal contraceptives, such as oral, intravaginal, or intrauterine, for the treatment of primary dysmenorrhea is limited, although this

Table 2
Formulations and recommended dosages of nonsteroidal anti-inflammatory drugs

Agent	Loading Dose	Maintenance Dose[a]
Ibuprofen	400 mg	200–400 mg q 4–6 h
Naproxen	500 mg	250 q 6°–8° or 500 q 12°
Naproxen sodium	550 mg	275 mg q 6°–8° or 550 mg q 12°
Diclofenac potassium	100 mg	50 q 6°–8° (max daily dose 200 mg)
Mefenamic acid	500 mg	250 q 6° or 500 mg q 8°

[a] Recommended for duration of menses or as long as pain is experienced.

is common clinical practice, especially for dysmenorrhea that is unresponsive to initial treatment with NSAIDs.[19] High-quality randomized clinical trials evaluating the effectiveness of oral contraceptives in reducing menstrual pain are lacking, although smaller studies have found response rates as high as 80%.[20]

Combined hormonal contraceptives, including combined oral contraceptives, the contraceptive ring, and the transdermal patch, all work to decrease the endometrial lining, which in itself produces prostaglandins and leukotrienes that contribute to the menstrual pain. In addition, their role in inhibiting ovulation and subsequent progesterone production also decreases the formation of prostaglandins and leukotrienes. Thus, these products have been prescribed for primary dysmenorrhea, as well as some causes of secondary dysmenorrhea, particularly endometriosis. Davis and colleagues[21] demonstrated in a randomized clinical trial that adolescents with moderate and severe dysmenorrhea experienced reduced pain with a cyclic prescribed low-dose combined oral contraceptive (levonorgestrel 100 mgs plus ethinyl estradiol 20 μg). Reports of pain relief have also been greater with the vaginal ring than the transdermal patch and some studies have found menstrual pain exacerbated with the patch.[13,22] In a small randomized clinical trial with 35 adolescents and young adults, continuous combined oral contraceptives showed more immediate relief of pain than cyclic contraceptive pills, although the effects were similar at 6 months.[23] Given that an adolescent may abandon a method if no relief is experienced within 2 to 3 menstrual cycles, continuous methods may be preferable. The effectiveness of extended, continuous cycles has also been described using the vaginal ring.[24] Keep in mind that with the sexually active adolescent, the use of hormonal contraception for management of the dysmenorrhea also provides effective contraception.

Long-acting reversible contraceptives have also been found to be effective treatments for both primary and secondary dysmenorrhea. These include the levonorgestrel-containing intrauterine system, LNG-IUS (Mirena), the etonogestrel-containing subdermal implant (Nexplanon), and depot-medroxyprogesterone. For the sexually active adolescent, these also provide the benefit of highly effective contraception. Concerns about the long-term adverse effect of medroxyprogesterone on bone accretion and weight gain need to be considered. In a study from the United Kingdom, 92% of adolescents reported significant improvements in menstrual pain with the LNG-IUS.[25] Another study by Subhonen and colleagues[26] reported better efficacy of the LNG-IUS compared with combined oral contraceptives. The etonogestrel-containing subdermal implant has also been shown to have similar efficacy to the LNG-IUS, with 81% reporting improvement in menstrual pain.[27] Endometrial atrophy caused by the LNG-IUS and the inhibition of ovulation caused by both depot medroxyprogesterone and the etonogestrel implant have been postulated as mechanisms accounting for their beneficial effect on menstrual pain.

Nonpharmacologic Treatment Options

Several studies have assessed the role of complementary alternative and nonpharmacological therapies for the treatment of primary dysmenorrhea. Khan and colleagues[28] examined several systematic reviews and trials evaluating the efficacy of nondrug, nonsurgical treatments for primary dysmenorrhea. They found that, although many of these interventions, such as acupressure, behavioral therapies, herbal remedies, thiamine, transcutaneous electrical nerve stimulation, topical heat, and Vitamin E, have some evidence of effectiveness, the strength of this effectiveness is very weak and the quality of the studies in general were poor. They concluded that good quality and more creative and innovative research in this area is needed to guide clinical practice for these methods.

Treatment of Secondary Dysmenorrhea

If the history and physical examination point to a pathologic cause for the dysmenorrhea, the diagnostic evaluation can be tailored to the specific condition under consideration and treatment provided for that condition (see **Table 1**). In addition, if primary dysmenorrhea is initially suspected and the adolescent fails to respond to treatment with either an NSAID or hormonal treatment after 2 to 3 full menstrual cycles, consideration of less common causes for dysmenorrhea are imperative.

For endometriosis, combined oral contraceptives are recommended as the first-line treatment and have been found to be highly effective.[29] In addition, several clinical trials have supported the use of depot medroxyprogesterone, the etonogestrel subdermal implant (Nexplanon), and the LNG-IUS (Mirena) in endometriosis.[30] Laufer and colleagues[31] found that in a group of adolescents who reported lack of response to either NSAIDs or combined hormonal contraceptives, a 67% rate of endometriosis was diagnosed through laparoscopy. Delay in diagnosis in adolescents has also been attributed to the fact that they may report noncyclic pain and may lack the experiences of dyspareunia or fertility problems.

With any müllerian anomaly that presents with cyclic pain, as well as menses, the assumption is that there is partial patency of the uterine or vaginal tracts. In the case of obstructing uterine horns or vaginal septa, referral to a gynecologist for surgical repair is indicated. The reader is referred to the excellent references published by Dietrich for a full description of these müllerian anomalies.[16,17]

ADDITIONAL CONSIDERATIONS

As previously described, most cycles in the first 2 years after menarche are anovulatory.[1] Despite this lack of ovulation, regular menses are possible in response to the cyclic rising and falling levels of estrogen secreted from developing follicles that cause endometrial lining buildup followed by periodic shedding. In fact, a prospective study from the WHO of early adolescent girls found that by 2 years after menarche, 67% of menstrual cycles were reported as regular (ie, occurring at intervals of 20–40 days and lasting no more than 10 days) and, presumably, many of these regular menses were anovulatory.[32] Further, this study also found that 5% of these young adolescents reported cycles lasted longer than 7 days, and 0.5% longer than 10 days. Thus, it is relatively uncommon for these anovulatory cycles secondary to an immature H-P-G axis to result in an unstable endometrium that produces irregular sloughing and excessive of prolonged uterine bleeding.[33]

However, there may be specific pathologic conditions in which menarche is associated with excessive uterine bleeding requiring evaluation and treatment. These conditions encompass a wide variety of causes, and the pathophysiology associated with each depends on whether it is hormonally mediated, secondary to a systemic medical condition, arising from a specific genital tract abnormality, or pregnancy-associated. If excessive bleeding during cyclic menses is associated with signs of ovulation, such as cramping, premenstrual, or systemic symptoms, the cause is more likely to be either normal bleeding perceived as excessive by the teen or a bleeding diathesis. With cyclic or noncyclic bleeding that is painless, anovulatory bleeding should be suspected and a variety of hormonally mediated conditions that cause disruption of the H-P-G axis are more likely to be involved. A complete discussion of these conditions is beyond the scope of this article. A situation that may arise at the outset of menarche is the excessive uterine bleeding secondary to a bleeding disorder.

Bleeding disorders are important conditions to consider with any adolescent presenting with excessive uterine bleeding, especially when it presents soon after menarche. Claessen and Cowell[34] reported on a series of adolescents presenting for acute menorrhagia and found that 20% overall, 25% of those with a presenting hemoglobin less than 10 mg/100 mL, and 50% of those presenting at menarche were subsequently found to have a primary coagulation disorder. Von Willebrand disease, a deficiency of clotting factors important in platelet adhesion, is the most commonly seen inherited coagulation disorder but others, such as hemophilia A or B, can be seen. Acquired platelet disorders can also present with menorrhagia and include idiopathic thrombocytopenia purpura, autoimmune disorders, and aplastic anemia, as well as congenital disorders such as Glanzmann thrombasthenia.[35]

Because excessive bleeding can cause hemodynamic instability and anemia, it is also essential for the pediatrician to determine the acuity versus chronicity of the bleeding, and probe for specific signs that indicate hypovolemia and/or anemia. These may indicate the need to determine volume status urgently, as a priority over determining the cause of the excessive bleeding. Symptoms of fatigue, light-headedness, presyncope should all raise concern about the teen's hemodynamic stability. In the setting of acute bleeding and/or hypovolemia, referral to an emergency setting and consultation with either a gynecologist or a hematologist are most appropriate.

REFERENCES

1. Hertweck SP. Dysfunctional uterine bleeding. Obstet Gynecol Clin North Am 1992;19:129.
2. Vihko R, Apter D. Endocrine characteristics of adolescent menstrual cycles: impact of early menarche. J Steroid Biochem 1984;20:231.
3. Slap GB. Menstrual disorders in adolescence. Best Pract Res Clin Obstet Gynaecol 2003;17:75.
4. Elford KJ, Spence JE. The forgotten female: Pediatric and adolescent gynecological concerns and their reproductive consequences. J Pediatr Adolesc Gynecol 2002;15:65.
5. Harlow SD, Ephross SA. Epidemiology of menstruation and its relevance to women's health. Epidemiol Rev 1995;17(2):265–86.
6. Latthe P, Latthe M, Say L, et al. WHO systematic review of prevalence of chronic pelvic pain: a neglected reproductive health morbidity. BMC Public Health 2006; 6:177.
7. Latthe P, Mignini L, Gray R, et al. Factors predisposing women to chronic pelvic pain: systematic review. BMJ 2006;332:749–55.

8. Ju H, Jones M, Mishra G. The prevalence and risk factors of dysmenorrhea. Epidemiol Rev 2014;36:104–13.
9. Lentz G, Lobo R, Gershenson D, et al. Comprehensive gynecology. Philadelphia: Mosby Elsevier; 2012.
10. Wang L, Wang X, Wang W, et al. Stress and dysmenorrhea: a population based prospective study. Occup Environ Med 2004;61(12):1021–6.
11. Hauksson A, Akerlund M, Melin P. Uterine blood flow and myometrial activity at menstruation, and the action of vasopressin and a synthetic antagonist. Br J Obstet Gynaecol 1988;95:898–904.
12. Pulkkinen MO. Prostaglandins and the non-pregnant uterus. The pathophysiology of primary dysmenorrhea. Acta Obstet Gynecol Scand Suppl 1983;113:63–7.
13. Allen LM, Nevin Lam AC. Premenstrual syndrome and dysmenorrhea in adolescents. Adolesc Med 2012;23:139–63.
14. Willman EA, Collins WP, Clayton SG. Studies in the involvement of prostaglandins in uterine symptomatology and pathology. Br J Obstet Gynaecol 1976;83:337.
15. Akerlund M. Vascularization of human endometrium. Uterine blood flow in healthy condition and in primary dysmenorrhea. Ann N Y Acad Sci 1994;734:47–56.
16. Dietrich JE. Obstructive müllerian anomalies. (A NASPAG clinical recommendation). J Pediatr Adolesc Gynecol 2014;27(6):396–402.
17. Dietrich JE. Non-obstructive müllerian anomalies (A NASPAG clinical recommendation). J Pediatr Adolesc Gynecol 2014;27(6):386–95.
18. Marjoribanks J, Proctor M, Farquhar C, et al. Nonsteroidal anti-inflammatory drugs for dysmenorrhea. Cochrane Database Syst Rev 2010;20(1):CD001751.
19. Wong CL, Farquhar C, Roberts H, et al. Oral contraceptive pill for primary dysmenorrhea. Cochrane Database Syst Rev 2009;(2):CD002120.
20. American College of Obstetricians and Gynecologists. ACOG practice bulletin no. 110: noncontraceptive uses of hormonal contraceptives. Obstet Gynecol 2010;115:206–18.
21. Davis AR, Westhoff C, O'Connell K, et al. Oral contraceptives for dysmenorrhea in adolescent girls: a randomized clinical trial. Obstet Gynecol 2005;106:97–104.
22. Harel Z, Riggs S, Vaz R, et al. Adolescents' experience with the combined estrogen and progestin transdermal contraceptive method Ortho Evra. J Pediatr Adolesc Gynecol 2005;18:85–90.
23. Dmitrovic R, Kunselman A, Legro R. Continuous compared with cyclic oral contraceptives for the treatment of primary dysmenorrhea. A randomized controlled trial. Obstet Gynecol 2012;119:1143.
24. Barreiros FA, Guazzelli CA, Barbosa R, et al. Extended regimens of the contraceptive vaginal ring: evaluation of clinical aspects. Contraception 2010;81:223–5.
25. Aslam N, Blunt S, Latthe P. Effectiveness and tolerability of levonorgestrel intrauterine system in adolescents. J Obstet Gynaecol 2010;30:489–91.
26. Subhonen S, Haukkamaa M, Jakobsson T, et al. Clinical performance of a levonorgestrel-releasing intrauterine system and oral contraceptives in young nulliparous women; a comparative study. Contraception 2004;69:407–12.
27. Funk S, Miller MM, Mishell DR Jr, et al. Safety and efficacy of Implanon, a single-rod implantable contraceptive containing etonogestrel. Contraception 2005;71:319–26.
28. Khan K, Champaneria R, Latthe P. How effective are non-drug, non-surgical treatments for primary dysmenorrhea? BMJ 2012;344:e3011.
29. Harada T, Momoeda M, Taketani Y, et al. Low-dose oral contraceptive pill for dysmenorrhea associated with endometriosis: a placebo-controlled, double-blind, randomized trial. Fertil Steril 2008;90:1583–8.

30. Leyland N, Casoer R, Laberge P, et al, SOGC. Endometriosis: diagnosis and management. J Obstet Gynaecol Can 2010;32:S1–32.
31. Laufer MR, Goitein L, Bush M, et al. Prevalence of endometriosis in adolescent girls with chronic pain not responding to conventional therapy. J Pediatr Adolesc Gynecol 1997;10:199–202.
32. World Health Organization multicenter study on menstrual and ovulatory patterns in adolescent girls. II. Longitudinal study of menstrual patterns in the early post-menarcheal period, duration of bleeding episodes and menstrual cycles. World Health Organization Task Force on Adolescent Reproductive Health. J Adolesc Health Care 1986;7:236–44.
33. Jamieson M. Disorders of menstruation in adolescent girls. Pediatr Clin North Am 2015;62:943–61.
34. Claessens E, Cowell C. Acute adolescent menorrhagia. Am J Obstet Gynecol 1981;139:277.
35. Philip CS. Platelets disorders in adolescents. J Pediatr Adolesc Gynecol 2010;23: S11–4.

Choosing the Right Oral Contraceptive Pill for Teens

 CrossMark

Anne Powell, MD

KEYWORDS

- Oral contraceptive pill (OCP) • Combined oral contraceptive (COC)
- Progestin-only contraceptive (POP) • Venous thromboembolism (VTE)
- US medical eligibility criteria (US MEC)

KEY POINTS

- Oral contraceptive pills provide effective and safe contraception for adolescents when taken correctly.
- Oral contraceptive pills include 2 broad categories: progestin-only pills (POPs) and combined oral contraceptives (COCs).
- COCs lead to an increased risk of venous thromboembolism (VTE), so clinicians should perform a thorough assessment of any contraindications to estrogen before prescribing.
- COCs provide many noncontraceptive health benefits, including treatment of dysmenorrhea, excessive uterine bleeding, acne, and polycystic ovary syndrome.

INTRODUCTION

In 1960, the first oral contraceptive pill (OCP), Enovid, was approved by the US Food and Drug Administration.[1] Since that time, OCPs available to US women have changed dramatically, with decreased hormone concentrations and increased variety in formulations. As detailed in other articles in this publication, the American Academy of Pediatrics and American College of Obstetricians and Gynecologists advocate that long-acting reversible contraceptives (LARCs) be recommended as first-line contraceptive options for sexually active adolescents[2] (See Suzanne Allen and Erin Barlow's article, "LARC Methods," in this issue). Although trends are shifting in terms of increasing LARC use, OCPs continue to be the most common form of prescription contraception accessed by US adolescents.[3]

Disclosure: The author has no financial or commercial relationships or interests to disclose. There were no funding sources for this article.
Division of Adolescent Medicine, University of Massachusetts Medical School, 55 Lake Avenue North, Worcester, MA 01655, USA
E-mail address: anne.powell@umassmemorial.org

TYPES OF ORAL CONTRACEPTIVE PILLS, MECHANISM OF ACTION, AND EFFICACY

There are 2 broad categories of OCPs: progestin-only pills (POPs) and combined oral contraceptives (COCs). POPs function primarily through thickening the cervical mucus and thereby preventing sperm penetration. In addition, POPs inhibit ovulation to variable degrees, reduce cilia activity in the fallopian tubes, and alter the endometrium.[1] COCs, which contain both estrogen and progesterone, function primarily though inhibiting ovulation via feedback in the hypothalamic-pituitary-ovarian axis and thickening cervical mucus. When discussing efficacy of OCPs, it is crucial to distinguish perfect use from typical use. There is a significant discrepancy between these rates due to challenges with patient adherence to daily dosing. With *perfect* use, oral contraceptives have a 0.3% failure rate in the first year of use[4]; however, with *typical* use, oral contraceptives have a failure rate of 8% in the first year of use.[4] Although OCPs offer excellent pregnancy protection with proper use, they do not offer protection from sexually transmitted infections (STIs). As such, all patients using OCPs for contraception should also be counseled to use condoms consistently for STI protection (See Zoon Wangu and Gale R. Burstein's article, "Adolescent Sexuality: Updates to the Sexually Transmitted Infection Guidelines," in this issue).

Both POPs and COCs require daily dosing; however, POPs require more exact dosing to maintain contraceptive efficacy. For adolescents, daily dosing in general can be problematic. When counseling an adolescent about OCPs for birth control, it is important for clinicians to speak openly with patients about the challenges of daily dosing and explore whether the adolescent feels that she is capable of adherence. Many adolescents find using an alarm in their cell phones to be a useful tool in helping them remember to take their pills. Because POPs require exact dosing in terms of the hour taken each day, most clinicians try to avoid this method as a primary form of birth control in adolescents. However, POPs may be the only option available for certain patients. With such patients, counseling must be very direct about the necessity of exact dosing, as well as the strong recommendation for consistent condom use, as both STI protection and back-up contraception.

ADDRESSING COMMON CULTURAL MYTHS ABOUT ORAL CONTRACEPTIVE PILLS

Many patients have preconceived notions about the efficacy, safety, and side effects of OCPs. It is very useful to explore a patient's current understanding and knowledge of OCPs before prescribing so that common cultural "myths" can be dispelled. A common myth is that taking OCPs will impair a patient's future fertility. Generally, OCPs do not adversely affect fertility. For most patients, menstrual cycles return promptly to the same pattern that existed before starting OCPs.[1] Some women may experience some delay before menstrual cycles resume, but most do not.

Some patients may be concerned because menstrual flow is lighter than usual than what they experienced before starting OCPs. Some patients think that menstrual blood is "backing up" in their bodies. It is helpful to educate such patients about how OCPs prevent excessive build-up of the uterine lining, so infrequent menses, or light menses, while on OCPs does not pose a health risk.

Many patients believe that OCPs lead to significant weight gain. For some patients, this is a major reason to avoid OCPs, so it is important to address this concern in the early stages of contraceptive counseling. Patients will be reassured to know that multiple double-blind studies have shown no association between low-dose COC use and weight gain.[5]

Patients may also hold the belief that birth control is "artificial" and unsafe, whereas pregnancy represents a natural, safe condition. It can be useful to educate such patients that negative health issues associated with being pregnant and postpartum are far more common than with OCPs.

DECIDING BETWEEN PROGESTIN-ONLY PILLS AND COMBINED ORAL CONTRACEPTIVES

COCs are generally favored over POPs as a form of contraception because of the strict dosing schedule required by POPs. When deciding if an adolescent is an appropriate candidate for COCs, it is necessary to determine if the patient has a contraindication to estrogen-containing medications. The Centers for Disease Control and Prevention (CDC) recently published updated guidelines regarding medical eligibility for contraceptive use. This document, the US Medical Eligibility Criteria for Contraceptive Use (US MEC), is designed to assist clinicians to counsel patients about contraceptive method choice[4] and was adapted from global guidance provided by the World Health Organization (WHO). The US MEC includes recommendations for using specific contraceptive methods in patients with specific medical conditions and can be accessed through the CDC Web site.

When assessing a patient's safety profile regarding use of COCs, much of the decision-making revolves around the increased risk of venous thromboembolism (VTE) associated with estrogen. The relative risk of VTE in patients taking COCs is 3 to 5 times higher than in women who are not taking COCs.[3] Certain patient characteristics, such as smoking and obesity, also contribute to increased VTE risk. Although the *relative* risk is increased, the *absolute* risk of VTE remains very low. Estimates regarding the prevalence of nonfatal VTE in the general population are highly variable. At baseline, a general estimate of a young, healthy woman's risk of developing a VTE is 4 of 100,000 women per year.[3] This risk increases to approximately 10 to 30 of 100,000 women per year when a patient is on a low-dose COC.[3] However, when explaining this increased risk to patients, it is important to remind them that the risk of VTE when on a COC is still much lower than the risk of a VTE during pregnancy. During pregnancy, a woman's risk of VTE increases to approximately 60 of 100,000 women per year.[3]

As detailed in the US MEC, the WHO classifies medical eligibility criteria for contraception into 4 main categories, summarized in **Table 1**.[4]

When prescribing a COC, it is important to screen for common category 3 and 4 conditions that may pose contraindications to estrogen use. A clinician should inquire about personal and family history of VTE, history of migraine with aura, and history of hypertension. Patients who have underlying thrombophilias, such as Factor V Leiden deficiency, are not appropriate candidates for COC therapy. Common category 3 and 4 conditions are summarized in **Table 2**. Please note that this list is not comprehensive; the US MEC has a more thorough description of medical contraindications to COC treatment.

Table 1	
World Health Organization categories of medical eligibility criteria for contraceptive use	
Category 1	Condition for which there is no medical restriction to use method
Category 2	Advantages of using contraceptive method generally outweigh the risks
Category 3	Theoretic or proven risks usually outweigh advantages of contraceptive method
Category 4	Unacceptable health risk if contraceptive method used

Table 2
Common category 3 and 4 medical conditions from 2016 US medical eligibility criteria recommendations for COC use

Category 3 conditions (use of method generally not recommended)	• Adequately controlled hypertension • Superficial venous thrombosis (acute or history) • History of deep venous thrombosis (DVT) with low-risk recurrence DVT/pulmonary embolism (PE) • Use of certain anticonvulsants • Antiretroviral (ARV) treatment with Fosamprenavir (all other ARVs are categories 1 and 2)
Category 4 conditions (health risk associated with using method is unacceptable)	• Known thrombogenic mutation • Acute DVT • History of DVT, higher risk of recurrent DVT/PE • Postpartum <21 d • Migraine with aura • Uncontrolled hypertension • Lupus with positive or unknown antiphospholipid antibody • Major surgery with prolonged immobilization • Hepatocellular adenoma • Personal history of stroke • Complicated valvular heart disease

SMOKING AND COMBINED ORAL CONTRACEPTIVE USE

In adolescents, smoking does not represent an absolute contraindication to using COCs. Smoking alone increases the risk of VTE and this effect is compounded by COC use. Smoking itself causes 1.4 to 3.3 times risk increase in VTE.[6] The combination of COC use and smoking compounds this risk further, leading to an 8.8 times risk increase in VTE.[6] In patients younger than 35, smoking is classified as a category 2 condition.[4] In patients ages 35 or older, smoking becomes a category 3 or 4 condition depending on the number of cigarettes smoked per day.[4] Adolescent patients who smoke should be counseled about the increased risk of VTE and smoking cessation should be encouraged.

PRESCRIBING THE PROGESTIN-ONLY PILL

If a patient has a medical contraindication to estrogen or wishes to avoid estrogen for personal reasons, there are several nonhormonal methods and progestin-only methods available. As detailed in other articles of this issue, intrauterine devices are available in nonhormonal and progestin-only forms. Also, Nexplanon and Depo-Provera are highly effective contraceptive methods that contain progesterone only (See article, "LARC Methods," in this issue). Patients who have medical contraindications to estrogen should be counseled about these other contraceptive methods. Alternatively, patients can be offered the POP.

Most clinicians try to avoid the use of the POP as a primary method of contraception due to difficulties many patients have with the exact daily dosing that this medication requires. POPs contain the active ingredient norethindrone at a concentration of

0.35 mg. The POP pack contains 28 days of *active* hormonal pills. Many patients are familiar with the traditional packaging of estrogen-containing COCs; most have 3 consecutive weeks of active hormonal pills followed by 7 days of placebo pills. Patients being prescribed a POP should be clearly counseled that these pills do not have a placebo week and it is crucial that they take every pill in a pack to maintain contraceptive efficacy. Common side effects of POPs include intermittent amenorrhea and irregular spotting. POPs also have several health benefits, including improved dysmenorrhea and possible protection against endometrial cancer.[1]

QUICK START METHOD

The "traditional" way to initiate OCP use was to advise a patient to wait until her menstrual period and then start the OCP. This method is problematic in that many adolescents have irregular menses. Waiting for the onset of menses could result in significant delay in starting the OCP and could lead to an undesired "window of opportunity" for unintended pregnancy. Such reasoning supports the use of the "quick start method." The quick start method applies to all types of OCPs, both POPs and COCs.

With the quick start method, the patient starts the OCP medication as soon as it is prescribed. In all sexually active patients, it is recommended to check a urine pregnancy test before giving an OCP prescription. If the pregnancy test is negative and the patient's last menstrual period (LMP) was within the past 5 days, the patient may start the OCP on the day the script is provided. Back-up contraception is not necessary in this situation, although condoms are always recommended for STI protection.[1]

If the patient's LMP was more than 5 days ago, urine pregnancy test negative, and she has NOT had unprotected intercourse since LMP, the OCP can be started that day. In this situation, patients require back-up contraception for the first week of OCP use.

If the patient's LMP was more than 5 days ago and she has had unprotected intercourse, then she should be counseled about the potential for an early pregnancy that would not necessarily be reflected in a urine pregnancy test. Use of a POP or COC is not associated with teratogenic effects or adverse pregnancy outcomes.[1] Therefore, even if pregnancy cannot be definitively excluded, patients can be given the option to start an OCP and return for follow-up pregnancy testing within 2 to 3 weeks. If a patient has had unprotected intercourse within the past 5 days, she should be offered emergency contraception (EC) (See Ellen S. Rome and Veronica Issac's article, "Emergency Contraception," in this issue). If she chooses, the patient should take EC as soon as possible and then start the OCP that same day. The patient should be advised to use back-up contraception for 1 week and should return for follow-up pregnancy testing in 2 weeks.

Some patients may not be comfortable starting a contraceptive method when pregnancy cannot be definitively excluded and do not choose EC. Such patients can be provided with a script for the OCP and advised to use barrier contraception until their next menses. Patients should be advised to start the OCP on the first day of menses or the first Sunday following menses and should also be encouraged to return for pregnancy testing if menses is late.

PRESCRIBING COMBINED ORAL CONTRACEPTIVES

Just as with POPs, the quick start method is effective. COCs contain both estrogen and progesterone and function primarily through inhibiting ovulation and thickening cervical mucus. Benefits and risks associated with COCs and differences among COC formulations are discussed in the following sections.

NONCONTRACEPTIVE HEALTH BENEFITS OF COMBINED ORAL CONTRACEPTIVES

In addition to providing birth control, COCs offer several other health benefits noted in **Table 3**. COCs can provide menstrual regulation, decreased menstrual flow, and improved dysmenorrhea. Many patients opt to use COCs for treatment of irregular, heavy, or painful menses (See Sheryl A. Ryan's article, "The Treatment of Dysmenorrhea and Excessive Uterine Bleeding," in this issue). COCs can help prevent and treat iron-deficiency anemia associated with menorrhagia. Long-term (>5 years) COC use offers some protective effects against endometrial and ovarian cancer.[7] COC use can prevent ovarian cyst formation due to inhibition of ovulation. Certain formulations improve acne and hirsutism, which are discussed later.

SIDE EFFECTS AND MEDICAL RISKS ASSOCIATED WITH COMBINED ORAL CONTRACEPTIVES

One of the most common side effects associated with COC use is irregular, breakthrough menstrual bleeding. Breakthrough bleeding (BTB) typically resolves within the first 3 cycles of COC use and patients should be counseled proactively about this possible side effect. Management of persistent BTB is discussed later. Some patients may experience nausea after taking COCs. For such patients, taking the COC with food or in the evening can be helpful.

Among the greatest concerns related to COC therapy is increased incidence of VTE. Risk of VTE is most prominent during the first year of use, particularly during the first 3 months of use.[3] Depending on the age and medical profile of the patient, other serious, but uncommon risks include myocardial infarction, stroke, hypertension, and benign liver tumors.[1] These side effects and medical risks are summarized in **Table 4**.

When initiating COC therapy, it is crucial to counsel patients about the increased VTE risk and educate them about concerning symptoms. The ACHES mnemonic may help patients remember symptoms related to VTE complications:

A bdominal pain
C hest pain
H eadaches
E ye symptoms (such as vision changes)
S evere leg pain

Table 3	
Noncontraceptive health benefits of combined oral contraceptives (COCs)	
Menstrual-related	• Improved dysmenorrhea • Decreased menstrual blood flow • Regulation of menstrual cycle • Reduction in premenstrual syndrome symptoms (PMS) • Reduction in premenstrual dysphoric disorder (PMDD) symptoms
Hematologic	• Decreased iron-deficiency anemia
Cancer prevention	• Decreased risk of endometrial cancer • Decreased risk of ovarian cancer
Dermatologic	• Improved acne (with certain COC formulations) • Improved hirsutism (with certain COC formulations)
Ovarian	• Prevention of ovarian cysts • Relief of Mittelschmerz (ovulatory pain)

| Table 4 |
Side effects and medical risks associated with combined oral contraceptive use
Common side effects	• Breakthrough bleeding • Intermittent amenorrhea • Nausea • Breast tenderness • Headaches
Serious medical risks	• Venous thromboembolism • Pulmonary embolus • Myocardial infarction • Stroke • Hypertension • Gallbladder disease • Cholestatic jaundice • Benign liver tumors • Melasma/chloasma (increased melanocyte activity, patchy facial discoloration) • Slight increase in risk of cervical dysplasia and cervical carcinoma

OBESITY AND COMBINED ORAL CONTRACEPTIVES

There has been increasing concern about the safety and efficacy of COCs in obese women. Women who are obese and taking estrogen are at even higher risk of VTE than are women with normal body mass index (BMI) who are taking comparable doses of estrogen. The US MEC classifies obesity as a category 2 condition for women of any age. Obese patients being prescribed COCs should be counseled that achieving a healthier BMI can help decrease their VTE risk.

Studies have been conflicting regarding whether or not COCs have slightly lower efficacy rates in obese women. Peak hormone concentrations achieved in obese women taking COCs have been found to be less than in women with BMIs in the normal range.[8] However, the potential differences in peak hormone levels have not been shown to affect breakthrough ovulation.[9] Several studies have suggested that obese women have higher failure rates of COCs.[10] Other studies have been reassuring that elevated BMI does not compromise COC efficacy.[11] The Society of Family Planning has concluded that overweight and obese patients using COCs appear to be at similar or slightly higher risk of pregnancy compared with women who have a normal-range BMI.[12]

Bariatric surgery is becoming more common in the adolescent population. History of bariatric surgery, both restrictive and malabsorptive procedures, is considered to be category 1 and does not pose a contraindication to COC use.[13]

BREAST CANCER RISK AND COMBINED ORAL CONTRACEPTIVES

The topic of whether the risk of breast cancer increases with COC use can be confusing. This question has been reviewed in the medical literature extensively. In a 2002 study published in the *New England Journal of Medicine*, current or former oral contraceptive use was found NOT to be associated with increased risk of breast cancer.[14] Similarly, a large-scale prospective study published in *Contraception* in 2013 found no association between oral contraceptive use and overall breast cancer risk.[13] The Collaborative Group on Hormonal Factors in Breast Cancer synthesized and reanalyzed the epidemiologic data on the relationship between COCs and breast cancer on a worldwide, large-scale level.[15] That group concluded that there is a small increase in the risk of having breast cancer diagnosed while taking COCs and in the

10 years after COC discontinuation.[15] Cancers diagnosed in this group tended to be much less clinically advanced than in women not taking COCs.[15] Results of the study also found, however, that there is no significantly excess risk of having breast cancer diagnosed in women more than 10 years after COC discontinuation.[15] In general, COCs are considered to be safe and effective in young women, even if there is a family history of breast cancer.[14]

MEDICATION INTERACTIONS AND COMBINED ORAL CONTRACEPTIVES

It is important to review all medications that a patient is taking to screen for potential medication interactions. A common misconception is that broad-spectrum antibiotics compromise the efficacy of COCs. It is true that antibiotics can alter hepatic metabolism and lead to decreased levels of circulating estrogen in patients taking COCs; however, this decreased estrogen level is not *clinically* significant in that it does not impair COC efficacy. The vast majority of antibiotics, antifungals, and antiparasitic medications are classified as category 1 (no medical restriction to use method). Exceptions to this are rifampin and rifabutin, which are classified as category 3 (risks generally outweigh benefits).

Certain anticonvulsants, some of which are also used as mood stabilizers, can interact negatively with COCs and compromise COC efficacy. These include phenytoin, barbiturates, carbamazepine, primidone, topiramate, and oxcarbazepine.[4] Also, it is notable that pharmacokinetic studies show that levels of lamotrigine decrease significantly with concurrent COC use.[4] For a patient taking lamotrigine (Lamictal) as a monotherapy for seizure disorders, COC use would not be recommended. **Table 5** summarizes the US eligibility criteria for commonly used medications.[4]

DIFFERENCES AMONG COMBINED ORAL CONTRACEPTIVE FORMULATIONS

In the United States, COC formulations differ in the following ways: (1) estrogen concentration, (2) type and concentration of progesterone, (3) monophasic versus multiphasic formulations, and (4) ratio of inactive to active hormonal pills.

Table 5	
Common medications and combined oral contraceptive use	
Broad-spectrum antibiotics	Category 1
Antifungal medications	Category 1
Antiparasitic medications	Category 1
Rifampin or rifabutin therapy	Category 3
Certain anticonvulsants • Phenytoin • Barbiturates • Carbamazepine • Oxcarbazepine • Primidone • Topiramate • Lamotrigine	Category 3
St John's Wart	Category 2
Selective serotonin reuptake inhibitors	Category 1
Antiretroviral therapy EXCEPT for fosamprenavir	Categories 1 and 2
Antiretroviral Therapy with fosamprenavir	Category 3

The 2 types of estrogen available in COC formulations are ethinyl estradiol and mestranol. Mestranol is available in a few 50 μg COCs and is uncommonly used; these pills are discussed in this article. COCs containing ethinyl estradiol (EE) are far more commonly used. Concentrations of EE in COCs range from 10 to 50 μg. Most COCs contain 20 to 35 μg of estrogen and there is only 1 COC available that has 10 μg of EE. In general, it is recommended to initiate COC treatment with a dose of EE that is in the 20-μg to 35-μg range. Doses of EE greater than 35 μg are associated with higher risk of VTE.

Variations in estrogen concentrations in the 10-μg to 35-μg range lead to differences in other side effects. Lower-estrogen pills are associated with decreased levels of nausea, gastrointestinal upset, and breast tenderness, but can be associated with higher levels of breakthrough bleeding.[1] So, for a patient with heavy menstrual bleeding, a clinician would favor a COC pill with 30 to 35 μg of estrogen. Conversely, for a patient with a sensitive stomach concerned about nausea, a clinician would favor a COC pill with 20 μg of estrogen.

COMBINED ORAL CONTRACEPTIVES AND PROGESTINS

COCs differ in the concentration and type of progestin in their formulations. Progestins vary in terms of prothrombotic effect, potency of endometrial stabilization, and antiandrogenic activity. When selecting a COC for a particular patient, it is useful to match certain patient characteristics with specific progestin effects. Patient characteristics to consider include history of excessive uterine bleeding, acne, hirsutism, and polycystic ovary syndrome (PCOS). The types of progestins in COCs are norethindrone, levonorgestrel, norgestrel, desogestrel, and drospirenone.

PROGESTINS AND CLOTTING RISK

The VTE risk associated with COCs is related primarily to effects of estrogen. In recent years, there has been controversy in the medical community and the media about the possibility of certain progestins leading to increased clotting risk. COCs containing desogestrel include product labeling with information about a potential increased risk of VTE. This warning was based on international studies from the 1990s that suggested COCs containing desogestrel were associated with a higher VTE risk than COCs containing levonorgestrel and norgestrel.[16] Validity of these results is controversial and desogestrel-containing COCs remain widely prescribed.[1] However, more recent studies support the finding that desogestrel-containing COCs are associated with relatively increased risk of VTE compared with levonorgestrel-containing pills.[6]

There has also been controversy about the safety of the progestin drospirenone. Studies have been conflicting about whether drospirenone is associated with elevated VTE risk compared with levonorgestrel. A recent Cochrane Systematic Review article concluded that, as expected, all COCs investigated were associated with an increased risk of VTE.[17] However, the risk of VTE was found to vary depending on type of progestin. COCs containing desogestrel and drospirenone were associated with an approximately 50% to 80% higher VTE risk than with levonorgestrel-containing COCs.[17] But the *absolute* risk of VTE associated with COCs with these progestin components remains low and desogestrel and drospirenone remain widely prescribed.

PROGESTINS AND ANTIANDROGENIC EFFECTS

Certain progestin components have stronger antiandrogenic properties than others. Antiandrogenic effects are useful in treating patients with acne, hirsutism, and/or

PCOS. Progestins that have strong antiandrogenic benefits are norgestimate, drospirenone, and desogestrel. This is summarized in **Fig. 1**.

CHOOSING AN INITIAL COMBINED ORAL CONTRACEPTIVE FOR PATIENTS WITHOUT EXCESSIVE UTERINE BLEEDING, ACNE, HIRSUTISM, OR POLYCYSTIC OVARY SYNDROME

In patients who require only contraception and/or dysmenorrhea, it is not necessary to start with an antiandrogenic progestin. The progestins norethindrone, levonorgestrel, and norgestrel are all appropriate in this patient profile. Estrogen concentration should be started at a concentration of 35 μg or less. Some common COCs that contain the aforementioned progestins and also have 35 μg or less of estrogen are listed in **Table 6**.

CHOOSING AN INITIAL COMBINED ORAL CONTRACEPTIVE FOR PATIENTS WITH MENORRHAGIA AND/OR EXCESSIVE UTERINE BLEEDING

When selecting a COC for a patient with menorrhagia and/or excessive uterine bleeding, the priority is to stabilize the endometrium and cease bleeding as quickly and safely as possible. The progestin norgestrel is highly effective at stabilizing the endometrium. Oral contraceptives with this progestin are excellent choices for patients with menorrhagia. In patients with menorrhagia, patients can often benefit from having fewer menstrual periods per year. COCs can be prescribed to provide continuous cycling, which is discussed further later in this article. In patients who have menorrhagia and/or excessive bleeding but also need antiandrogenic effects for treatment of acne and PCOS, a clinician should opt for a norgestimate-containing COC.

CHOOSING AN INITIAL COMBINED ORAL CONTRACEPTIVE FOR PATIENTS WITH ACNE, HIRSUTISM, AND/OR POLYCYSTIC OVARY SYNDROME

Patients with acne, hirsutism and/or PCOS benefit from COCs that offer a combination of antiandrogenic effect, menstrual regulation, and contraception. The progestins norgestimate, desogestrel, and drospirenone all offer strong antiandrogenic properties. COCs with antiandrogenic progestins are summarized in **Table 7**. As discussed, the potential for increased clotting risk with drospirenone and desogestrel remains controversial. Norgestimate is a progestin that offers excellent antiandrogenic effect with a VTE risk that has been consistently shown to be similar to levonorgestrel.[6] In initial selection of a COC for a patient needing strong antiandrogen effect, it is very reasonable to select a norgestimate-containing pill. **Fig. 2** summarizes the basic approach to choosing an initial OCP depending on patient characteristics.

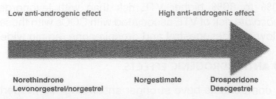

Low anti-androgenic effect   High anti-androgenic effect

Norethindrone   Norgestimate   Drosperidone
Levonorgestrel/norgestrel   Desogestrel

Fig. 1. Progestins and antiandrogenic properties.

Table 6
Common combined oral contraceptives (COCs) containing norethindrone, levonorgestrel, and norgestrel categorized by concentration of ethinyl estradiol (EE)

	35 μg EE	30 μg EE	20–25 μg EE
Norethindrone-containing COCs	Ortho-Novum 1/35 Necon 0.5/35	Lo-estrin 1/5/30 Junel 1.5/30 Microgestin 1/5/30	Lo-estrin 1/20 Junel 1/20 Microgestin 1/20
Levonorgestrel-containing COCs		Nordette Portia Levlen Levora Seasonale Quasense Jolessa	Aviane Alesse
Norgestrel-containing COCs		Lo-Ovral Cryselle Low-Ogestrel	

MONOPHASIC VERSUS MULTIPHASIC COMBINED ORAL CONTRACEPTIVE FORMULATIONS

In monophasic COCs, there is the same concentration of estrogen and progesterone in every active hormonal pill in the pack. In contrast, concentrations of hormone vary over the course of the pill pack in multiphasic formulations. There are no benefits associated with multiphasic COCs compared with monophasic COCs with comparable hormone concentrations.[18]

EXTENDED AND CONTINUOUS CYCLING

For both personal and medical reasons, minimizing the number of menses per year is highly desirable for many women. Certain menstrual-related medical issues, such as dysmenorrhea, endometriosis, premenstrual dysphoric disorder (PMDD), and menorrhagia, can be helped by reducing the number of cycles per year. Although some

Table 7
Common COCs containing norgestimate, desogestrel, and drospirenone categorized by concentration of ethinyl estradiol (EE)

	20 μg EE	30 μg EE	35 μg EE
Norgestimate-containing COCs			Ortho-cyclen Sprintec MonoNessa Previfem
Desogestrel-containing COCs	Mircette Kariva Mercilon	Desogen Reclipsen Ortho-cept Apri	
Drospirenone-containing COCs	YAZ BEYAZ Gianvi Vestura Yasminelle	Yasmin Zarah Ocella Safyral	

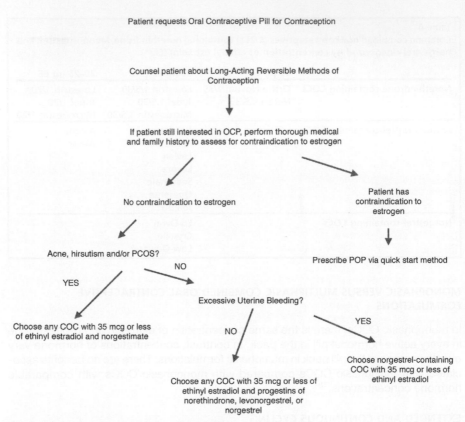

Patient requests Oral Contraceptive Pill for Contraception

Counsel patient about Long-Acting Reversible Methods of Contraception

If patient still interested in OCP, perform thorough medical and family history to assess for contraindication to estrogen

No contraindication to estrogen

Patient has contraindication to estrogen

Acne, hirsutism and/or PCOS?

YES   NO

Prescribe POP via quick start method

Choose any COC with 35 mcg or less of ethinyl estradiol and norgestimate

Excessive Uterine Bleeding?

NO   YES

Choose norgestrel-containing COC with 35 mcg or less of ethinyl estradiol

Choose any COC with 35 mcg or less of ethinyl estradiol and progestins of norethindrone, levonorgestrel, or norgestrel

Fig. 2. Algorithm for choosing an initial COC.

patients may feel reassured by having a monthly menses, there is no *medical* reason why patients need to have monthly withdrawal bleeds while taking COCs. Extended and continuous cycling with COCs is safe and effective. Safety profile and efficacy rates are comparable among cyclic, continuous, and extended cycling COC use.[19] A recent Cochrane Review found that, in 11 of the 12 studies examined, bleeding patterns were equivalent among cyclic, continuous, and extended cycling groups.[19]

Certain formulations of COCs are packaged with a higher ratio of active to inactive pills. For example, in Seasonale and its generic equivalents, there are 84 active pills and 7 inactive pills. Such formulations allow for patients to have a menstrual period approximately 4 times per year. Any monophasic COC formulation can be manipulated to provide extended cycling. If a traditional 28-day COC is prescribed and a patient requires or desires extended cycling, the patient is instructed to take the active hormonal pills for 3 weeks, discard the placebo week, and proceed directly to the next pack. When prescribed in this way, it can be useful for the prescription to indicate that the patient should be provided 2 packs as a 1 month supply. Patients may elect to have a "scheduled" withdrawal bleed every few months, which means they would take the placebo week every third or fourth pill pack if desired.

With continuous cycling, the patient takes active hormonal pills daily without any scheduled withdrawal bleeding. Lybrel is a COC that is designed specifically for continuous cycling. Lybrel contains 90 μg levonorgestrel and 20 μg EE per pill with no inactive pills. Similar to extended cycling, patients may also use any monophasic

COC formulation to provide continuous cycling. Patients simply take the active pills continuously, skipping the placebo week, until menstrual bleeding occurs. Once bleeding occurs, the patient allows a pill-free interval between 3 and 7 days and then resumes taking continuous active pills.

GENERAL FOLLOW-UP AND TROUBLESHOOTING SIDE EFFECTS

After starting on OCPs, patients should be seen for follow-up within 3 months to check up on medication adherence and side effects. Blood pressure should be monitored and STI testing may also be considered. Clinicians should inquire about the development of migraine headaches with aura or neurologic symptoms, which is an indication to discontinue estrogen use. Also, the "ACHES" symptoms associated with VTE should be reviewed.

Nausea and breast tenderness are common side effects associated with COC use. Typically, these side effects resolve within the first few cycles of use. If nausea and/or breast tenderness persist, clinicians may consider switching to a lower-estrogen COC formulation.

One of the most common side effects associated with COC use is BTB. Patients should be counseled proactively that BTB is very common during the first few months of COC use. It is not uncommon for adolescents to overestimate the severity of their menstrual blood loss. It may be useful to check a patient's hemoglobin and hematocrit when the degree of menstrual bleeding is in question. It is not recommended to switch a COC formulation solely in response to BTB within the first 3 cycles, unless the patient finds the side effect completely intolerable or unless there is true menorrhagia and/or anemia associated with COC use. In general, light to moderate BTB typically resolves after 3 months of COC use.

If BTB persists after 3 months, clinicians have several options to offer patients. If a patient is on an OCP with an estrogen concentration less than 35 μg, then increasing the dose of estrogen may help to stabilize the endometrium. If the dose of estrogen is already maximized at 35 μg, then the COC formulation can be changed to a more potent progestin component. Progestins that are particularly potent in terms of stabilizing the endometrium include norgestrel and norgestimate.

MANAGING MISSED PILLS

Missing pills is a very common occurrence, and patients should be counseled proactively about how to handle this situation. Recommendations on how to manage missed pills vary in level of complexity and can at times be difficult for patients to understand. The most recent edition of Contraceptive Technology offers a simplified approach to managing missed pills, which is summarized in **Table 8**.[1]

MANAGING PILL DOSING WITH VOMITING AND/OR DIARRHEA

If a patient vomits within 2 hours of taking a COC, she should proceed as if the pill were missed and use back-up contraception until she has had 7 days of taking active pills successfully.[1] Similarly, if a patient has severe vomiting and diarrhea for 2 days or more, she should be managed as if pills were missed.[1]

PATIENTS WITH CHRONIC MEDICAL CONDITIONS AND COMBINED ORAL CONTRACEPTIVE USE

Adolescents with chronic medical issues require special care and consideration when it comes to contraception. Many chronic medical issues, such as cystic fibrosis (CF),

Table 8
Simplified management of missed pills

	Catch-up Dosing	Emergency Contraception (EC)?	Back-up Contraception?
Missed 1 pill, <12 h late	• Take missed pill ASAP • Resume usual dosing	Not needed	Not needed
Missed 1 pill, >12 h late	• Take missed pill ASAP • Resume usual dosing	Not needed	Yes, condoms or abstinence × 7 d
Missed 2 or more pills, has at least 7 active pills remaining in pill pack	• Take forgotten pill and today's pill (2 pills on same day) • Resume usual dosing	Take EC if unprotected intercourse in past 7 d	Yes, condoms or abstinence × 7 d
Missed 2 or more pills, has 7 or fewer active pills remaining in pack: OPTION 1	• Take forgotten pill and today's pill (2 pills on same day) • Resume usual dosing	Take EC if unprotected intercourse in past 7 d	Yes, condoms or abstinence until she has taken 7 active pills in the NEXT PACK
Missed 2 or more pills, has 7 or fewer active pills remaining in pack: OPTION 2	• Take forgotten pill and today's pill (2 pills on same day) • Take the rest of the *active* pills in the pack • Skip placebo pills and proceed directly to next pack	Take EC if unprotected intercourse in past 7 d	Yes, condoms or abstinence × 7 d

Adapted from Hatcher RA. Contraceptive technology. New York: Ardent Media; 2011.

are associated with increased risk of adverse health events as a result of pregnancy, making effective contraception especially important. Some chronic medical issues, such as migraine headaches with aura, place patients at increased risk of medical complications associated with estrogen use. As such, clinicians should consult up-to-date guidelines in the US MEC when prescribing contraception to adolescents with chronic health conditions. The relationship between select common chronic health issues in adolescents and COC use is discussed in this section.

In the most recent US MEC guidelines, CF is classified as a category 1 condition with regard to COC use[4]; however, patients with CF are at increased risk of liver disease, gallbladder disease, and VTE associated with central venous catheters. The safety categories assigned to these other medical conditions are the same as for women who do not have CF. The category 1 classification for CF is based on the assumption that these other medical conditions are NOT present. Furthermore, certain medications used to treat CF can decrease the effectiveness of COCs, so clinicians should check potential medication interactions before prescribing a COC to a patient with CF.

Infection with human immunodeficiency virus (HIV) is classified as a category 1 condition. As with CF, a clinician should consider the potential for medication interaction when prescribing COCs to a patient with HIV. Most antiretroviral medications are classified as categories 1 or 2, making COCs an appropriate choice for most patients with HIV.[4] However, the antiretroviral agent fosamprenavir (FPV) is classified as category 3, and COCs should be avoided in in patients taking FPV.[4]

For most adolescent patients with insulin-dependent and non–insulin-dependent diabetes mellitus (DM), COCs are classified as category 2, making COCs an appropriate option for teens with DM.[4] However, if patients with DM also have neuropathy, retinopathy, other vascular disease, or have had DM for more than 20 years, the safety classification for COCs changes to categories $^3/_4$.[4]

In patients with inflammatory bowel disease (IBD), COCs are classified as categories 2/3. For patients with IBD and no other risk factors for VTE, COC use is considered category 2 and benefit generally outweighs the risks. However, in patients with IBD and an increased risk of VTE, such as extensive disease, surgery, and/or immobilization, COCs change to category 3 and risks generally outweigh benefits.[20] In patients with mild ulcerative colitis and no or small ileal resection, absorption of COCs appears intact.[20] It is possible that absorption may be impaired in patients with Crohn disease or extensive bowel resection.[20] LARCs are classified as category 1 for patients with IBD and may provide a safe and effective alternative for teen patients with IBD.[4]

For patients with systemic lupus erythematosus (SLE), safety classification for COC use depends on whether the patient has antiphospholipid antibodies. In patients with SLE who have positive or unknown antiphospholipid antibodies, COCs are classified as category 4 and represent an unacceptable health risk.[4] For patients with SLE and negative antiphospholipid antibodies, COCs are classified as category 2.[4]

REFERRING TO ADOLESCENT MEDICINE OR GYNECOLOGY

Many primary care providers are comfortable managing OCPs in uncomplicated adolescent patients. In certain situations, it may be advisable to have an adolescent medicine specialist or gynecologist involved. Referrals to subspecialists should be considered in patients with structural gynecologic anomalies, patients with menorrhagia that has caused anemia, and in patients with complicated medical comorbidities. Patients with known or suspected endometriosis may benefit from establishing a long-term relationship with a gynecologist. Subspecialty consultation also may be considered in patients who have persistent side effects or BTB on OCP treatment.

SUMMARY

In summary, OCPs provide effective and safe contraception for adolescents when taken correctly. OCPs include 2 broad categories: POPs and COCs. Both POPs and COCs require daily dosing, although POPs require more exact dosing to maintain efficacy. Daily dosing can be challenging for adolescents, and strategies to improve adherence should be discussed proactively. COCs lead to an increased risk of VTE, so clinicians should perform a thorough assessment of any contraindications to estrogen before prescribing. The US MEC provides comprehensive guidelines about which contraceptive methods are appropriate for patients depending on their medical profiles. COCs provide many noncontraceptive health benefits, including treatment of dysmenorrhea, excessive uterine bleeding, acne, and PCOS. All sexually active adolescents should be counseled to use condoms consistently for prevention of STIs.

REFERENCES

1. Hatcher RA. Contraceptive technology. New York: Ardent Media; 2011.
2. Committee on Adolescent Health Care Long-Acting Reversible Contraception Working Group, The American College of Obstetricians and Gynecologists. Committee opinion no. 539: adolescents and long-acting reversible contraception: implants and intrauterine devices. Obstet Gynecol 2012;120(4):983–8.
3. Emans SJH, Laufer MR. Emans, Laufer, Goldstein's pediatric and adolescent gynecology. Philadelphia: Lippincott, Williams and Wilkins; 2012.

4. Curtis KM, Tepper NK, Jatlaoui TC, et al. U.S. Medical Eligibility Criteria for Contraceptive Use, 2016. MMWR Recomm Rep 2016;65(3):1–103.
5. Kharbanda EO, Parker ED, Sinaiko AR, et al. Initiation of oral contraceptives and changes in blood pressure and body mass index in healthy adolescents. J Pediatr 2014;165(5):1029–33.
6. Trenor CC, Chung RJ, Michelson AD, et al. Hormonal contraception and thrombotic risk: a multidisciplinary approach. Pediatrics 2011;127(2):347–57.
7. Hannaford PC, Selvaraj S, Elliott AM, et al. Cancer risk among users of oral contraceptives: cohort data from the Royal College of General Practitioner's oral contraception study. BMJ 2007;335(7621):651.
8. Westhoff CL, Torgal AH, Mayeda ER, et al. Pharmacokinetics of a combined oral contraceptive in obese and normal-weight women. Contraception 2010;81(6):474–80.
9. Westhoff CL, Torgal AH, Mayeda ER, et al. Ovarian suppression in normal-weight and obese women during oral contraceptive use: a randomized controlled trial. Obstet Gynecol 2010;116(2 Pt 1):275–83.
10. Holt VL, Cushing-Haugen KL, Daling JR. Body weight and risk of oral contraceptive failure. Obstet Gynecol 2002;99(5 Pt 1):820–7.
11. Kaneshiro B, Edelman A, Carlson N, et al. The relationship between body mass index and unintended pregnancy: results from the 2002 National Survey of Family Growth. Contraception 2008;77(4):234–8.
12. Society of Family Planning, Higginbotham S. Contraceptive considerations in obese women: release date 1 September 2009, SFP Guideline 20091. Contraception 2009;80(6):583–90.
13. Vessey M, Yeates D. Oral contraceptive use and cancer: final report from the Oxford-Family Planning Association contraceptive study. Contraception 2013;88(6):678–83.
14. Marchbanks PA, McDonald JA, Wilson HG, et al. Oral contraceptives and the risk of breast cancer. N Engl J Med 2002;346(26):2025–32.
15. Breast cancer and hormonal contraceptives: further results. Collaborative Group on Hormonal Factors in Breast Cancer. Contraception 1996;54(3 Suppl):1S–106S.
16. Spitzer WO, Lewis MA, Heinemann LA, et al. Third generation oral contraceptives and risk of venous thromboembolic disorders: an international case-control study. Transnational research group on oral contraceptives and the health of young women. BMJ 1996;312(7023):83–8.
17. de Bastos M, Stegeman BH, Rosendaal FR, et al. Combined oral contraceptives: venous thrombosis. Cochrane Database Syst Rev 2014;(3):CD010813.
18. Van Vliet HA, Grimes DA, Helmerhorst FM, et al. Biphasic versus monophasic oral contraceptives for contraception. Cochrane Database Syst Rev 2006;(3):CD002032.
19. Edelman A, Micks E, Gallo MF, et al. Continuous or extended cycle vs. cyclic use of combined hormonal contraceptives for contraception. Cochrane Database Syst Rev 2014;(7):CD004695.
20. Curtis KM, Tepper NK, Marchbanks PA. U.S. medical eligibility criteria for contraceptive use, 2010. J Womens Health (Larchmt) 2011;20(6):825–8.

Long-Acting Reversible Contraception

An Essential Guide for Pediatric Primary Care Providers

Suzanne Allen, MSN, RN, CPNP-PC[a], Erin Barlow, MD[b,c],*

KEYWORDS

- Long-acting reversible contraception (LARC) • Intrauterine device
- Contraceptive implant • Adolescent • Confidentiality • Efficacy • Management
- Anticipatory guidance

KEY POINTS

- Long-acting reversible contraception (LARC) methods are now recommended as the first line of contraception for nulliparous adolescents by the American Academy of Pediatrics and American College of Obstetrics and Gynecology.
- Hormonal LARC methods work by blocking ovulation, thickening cervical mucus, and changing the lining of the uterus. Nonhormonal methods work by altering the environment in the endometrium and inhibiting the motility of sperm.
- LARC methods are the most effective contraceptive methods after abstinence.
- Even if primary care providers are not trained to insert LARCs, they can advise and counsel their patients about LARC methods if they have knowledge about the methods.

INTRODUCTION

Long-acting reversible contraception (LARC) methods are 20% more effective than traditional combined hormonal contraceptives (CHCs) and are recommended by the American Academy of Pediatrics and American College of Obstetrics and Gynecology as the first-line contraceptive choice for adolescent girls.[1,2] Large studies have shown that LARC use reduces unintended pregnancies, increases user

Neither author has disclosures of financial or commercial conflicts of interest to make.
[a] Division of Adolescent Medicine, Department of Pediatrics, U Mass Memorial Children's Medical Center, 55 Lake Avenue North, Worcester, MA 01655, USA; [b] Division of Adolescent Gynecology, Department of Obstetrics/Gynecology, U Mass Medical School, 55 Lake Avenue North, Worcester, MA 01655, USA; [c] Division of Pediatric, Department of Pediatrics, U Mass Medical School, 55 Lake Avenue North, Worcester, MA 01655, USA
* Corresponding author. Division of Adolescent Gynecology, Department of Obstetrics/Gynecology, U Mass Medical School, 55 Lake Avenue North, Worcester, MA 01655.
E-mail address: erin.barlow2@umassmemorial.org

Pediatr Clin N Am 64 (2017) 359–369
http://dx.doi.org/10.1016/j.pcl.2016.11.014
0031-3955/17/© 2016 Elsevier Inc. All rights reserved.

pediatric.theclinics.com

satisfaction, and prolongs duration of use for contraception.[3,4] Primary care providers (PCPs) are on the front line in providing access to contraception for adolescents; however, contraceptive options have changed dramatically in the past decade and PCPs may find contraceptive counseling challenging.[5] This article prepares the PCP with knowledge on safety, efficacy, eligibility, confidentiality, anticipatory guidance, how to find a LARC provider, and troubleshooting common side effects. With this information, the PCP will find contraceptive counseling concerning LARC both satisfying and effective.

DISCUSSION
Why Contraception for Adolescents?

Teen birth rates in the United States have been declining steadily in the past 25 years and the teen birth rate for 2015 (22 births/1000 girls 15–19 years) is the lowest level recorded in recent history[6]; however, even the low rate for 2015 is much higher than the rates observed in other developed countries.[6] The consequences of teen pregnancy are widespread, including health risks to the mother and child, socioeconomic impact, and public financial burden (see Heidi K. Leftwich and Marcus Vinicius Ortega Alves' article, "Adolescent Pregnancy," in this issue).

When a young woman has access to contraception, she can safely delay pregnancy so as to finish her education, pursue a career, and then become a mother when she is better prepared. Adolescents who do not use contraception at their first sexual encounter are twice as likely to become teenage mothers as those who did use a method of contraception.[7] Effective contraceptive counseling with a focus on LARC, access to all contraceptive methods, and an understanding of the right to access confidential contraception are paramount to reducing the number of unintended pregnancies in the adolescent population. **Table 1** briefly outlines available contraceptive methods.

Table 1
Contraceptive options for adolescent females

Method	Brand Name	Duration
Intrauterine device[a]	Mirena, Skyla, Liletta, Kyleena, Paraguard	3–10 y
Subdermal implant[a]	Nexplanon	3 y
Injectable	Depo-Provera	11–13 wk
Combined hormonal contraceptives	Pill, patch, vaginal ring	Daily, weekly, monthly

[a] LARC method.

The Contraceptive CHOICE project in St Louis provided more than 9000 women free education and access to all contraceptive options, including intrauterine devices (IUDs), subdermal implant, injection, pill, patch, and vaginal ring. When LARC methods were offered alongside traditional methods, 75% of women selected LARC. LARC use resulted in a significant reduction in unintended pregnancies, reduced abortion rates, increased user satisfaction with their contraceptive method, and longer duration of use over non-LARC methods.[3,4] Despite these results, fewer than 5% of teens on birth control are using LARC methods.[8] Adolescents are still significantly more likely to be using less-effective methods, such as condoms (21%) and the pill (47%) for contraception.[9] To decrease unintended pregnancies, LARC methods should be offered first to sexually active adolescents if there is no contraindication.

Long-Acting Reversible Contraception Methods: How They Work

As seen in **Table 2**, the primary subdermal implant available in the United States today is marketed by Merck as Nexplanon and has been available since 2011. Before 2011, the implant had been available as Implanon and Norplant. The current implant contains etonogestrel and provides contraception for 3 years. Nexplanon was updated from Implanon to include barium sulfate, making it detectable on radiographs and the applicator was improved for safer and easier insertion. **Fig. 1** shows the Nexplanon implant.

Table 2			
Subdermal implant			
Brand Name	**Duration**	**Efficacy**	**Expected Bleeding Pattern**
Nexplanon	3 y; can be removed and replaced at 3 y	0.05% failure rate	Variable, ranges from none to light spotting. Some users experience prolonged bleeding.

The contraceptive effect is achieved without the use of estrogen. The implant continually releases etonogestrel, a synthetic progestin, which prevents fertilization from occurring by blocking ovulation, thickening cervical mucus, and changing the lining of the uterus. The implant is immediately reversible on removal. Blood levels of etonogestrel were undetectable 7 days after removal and pregnancy has been reported as soon as 7 to 14 days from removal.[10]

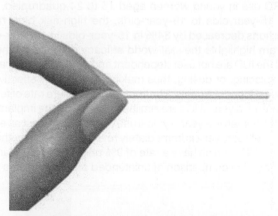

Fig. 1. Nexplanon. (NEXPLANON® image reproduced with permission of Merck Sharp & Dohme B.V., a subsidiary of Merck & Co., Inc., Whitehouse Station, New Jersey, USA. All rights reserved.)

Mirena, Skyla, Liletta, Kyleena, and Paraguard are the IUDs currently on the market for contraception. They are briefly compared in **Table 3**. The important difference to note among the 5 options is that the Paraguard copper IUD contains no hormones and contraception is achieved by copper changing the endometrium and inhibiting motility of sperm. Mirena, Skyla, Liletta, and Kyleena release levonorgestrel, which prevents pregnancy by preventing ovulation, thickening cervical mucus, promoting changes in the endometrium, and inhibiting motility of sperm.[11–14]

Table 3
Intrauterine devices (IUDs)

IUD Brand Name	Duration, y	Efficacy, % Failure Rate	Expected Bleeding Pattern
Mirena	5	0.2	None to light
Skyla	3	0.9	None to light
Liletta	3	0.2	None to light
Paraguard	10	0.8	Variable to heavy
Kyleena	5	<0.5	None to light

Mirena, Skyla, Liletta, and Kyleena lead to a reduction in menstrual flow over time. Mirena is also approved for treatment of dysmenorrhea. Menstrual bleeding is invariably heavier and longer in duration with Paraguard than with the levonorgestrel options; therefore, in most adolescent medicine settings, this is not a widely recommended option. However, Paraguard is the only IUD approved for emergency contraception and is 99.9% effective at preventing pregnancy if inserted within 5 days of unprotected intercourse.[11-14] Kyleena was approved for clinical use by the Food and Drug Administration in October 2016; therefore, additional data concerning its use among adolescent patients are still being gathered.

Why Long-Acting Reversible Contraception

Long-acting reversible contraception methods are the most effective contraceptive methods besides abstinence

In 2009, Colorado implemented full and free access to LARC methods for young women in the state's family planning clinics. Analysis of the outcomes of this program revealed that LARC use in young women aged 15 to 24 quadrupled, the fertility rate dropped 26% in 15-year-olds to 19-year-olds, the high-risk birth rate was greatly reduced, and abortions decreased by 34% in 15-year-olds to 19-year-olds.[15] The success of this program highlights the real-world efficacy of LARC methods.

The implant and the IUD are not user dependent and do not require maintenance, such as refills, timing, replacing, or dosing, thus making them highly effective contraceptive methods that are ideal for adolescents. The implant has a failure rate of fewer than 1 pregnancy per 100 women in a year. IUDs are similarly effective to the implant with fewer than 1 pregnancy per 100 women in a year. Typical use of LARC is at least as effective as many female sterilization methods, yet it is immediately reversible. LARC methods are 20 times more effective than CHCs, which have a rate of 9% unintended pregnancies per year.[16] See **Fig. 2** for side-by-side comparison of unintended pregnancy rates by method.

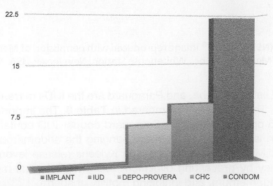

Fig. 2. Unintended pregnancy rate of contraceptive methods.

Long-acting reversible contraception methods are safe

IUDs are safe for nulliparous adolescents. Their use does not increase the risk for infection or infertility.[1,17] Appropriate screening must be done to rule out the possibility of current sexually transmitted infection (STI) before placement. If a patient is found to have an STI, the IUD cannot be inserted until after the infection has been treated. The IUD can remain in place without increased risk of developing pelvic inflammatory disease (PID) if the woman contracts an STI after placement. In fact, the presence of an IUD may lower the risk of acquiring PID secondary to the thickened cervical mucus and thinned out endometrial lining.[1,18] Prior use of currently available IUDs has not been associated with infertility.[1,17] Additionally, the contraceptive implant is safe and its use is associated with health benefits, including increased hemoglobin levels and reduction of dysmenorrheal and pelvic pain.[19–21]

Long-acting reversible contraception methods are approved for most adolescents

In addition to being the most effective forms of reversible contraception, LARC methods are also approved treatment for severe dysmenorrhea, endometriosis, heavy menstrual bleeding, and prevention of the development of ovarian cysts. The implant and IUD can be used to achieve menstrual suppression in adolescents who would benefit from suppression, such as those who are wheelchair bound or adolescents with developmental delays for whom personal hygiene at the time of menses presents a challenge.

There are far fewer contraindications to LARC use than contraceptives containing estrogen. Determining who is eligible for LARC is a straightforward process and the first step for the PCP when counseling the adolescent who is at risk for pregnancy and desires contraception. The nonpregnant, healthy adolescent with regular menstrual cycles is fully eligible with no contraindications.[22] LARC methods are safe for individuals who have contraindications for the use of CHCs, such as migraine with aura and history of deep vein thrombosis/pulmonary embolism (DVT/PE).[22] For IUD placement, the presence of an STI, such as PID or gonorrhea, is a contraindication to placement until the STI can be treated. Early pregnancy must be ruled out before placement or the patient must present for placement at the time of menses. Contraindications for LARC methods are listed in **Table 4**. For more in-depth information, a complete set of guidelines for use of various contraceptive agents, including LARC, can be found on the Centers for Disease Control and Prevention Web site: http://www.cdc.gov/reproductivehealth/contraception/usmec.htm.

Table 4
Contraindications for Initiating Use of Long-Acting Reversible Contraception Methods

Implant	Intrauterine Device
Unexplained vaginal bleeding	Unexplained vaginal bleeding
Acute deep vein thrombosis/pulmonary embolism (DVT/PE)	Acute DVT/PE
Systemic lupus erythematosus (SLE) with antiphospholipid antibodies	SLE with antiphospholipid antibodies
Severe cirrhosis, liver tumor	Severe cirrhosis, liver tumor
Current breast, ovarian, endometrial cancer	Current breast, ovarian, endometrial cancer
	Anatomic abnormalities of uterus
	Sexually transmitted infection, active

Adapted from World Health Organization (WHO). Medical eligibility criteria for contraceptive use. 5th edition. World Health Organization; 2015. Available at: http://www.who.int/reproductivehealth/publications/family_planning/Ex-Summ-MEC-5/en/.

Few drug interactions

Liver enzyme inducers, such as topiramate and lamotrigine, can speed up the metabolism of etonogestrel in the implant, which can contribute to decreased efficacy and breakthrough bleeding. These medications are not a contraindication to use, but users should be counseled on the potential for contraceptive failure and a backup method always should be used. If breakthrough bleeding continues and is bothersome, an IUD should be considered, as the hormone is absorbed locally and the drug interaction is decreased.[10]

Long-acting reversible contraception is affordable

Under the Affordable Care Act, LARC methods are covered by insurances as contraceptive methods. In the United States, low-income patients without insurance can access LARC methods at government-funded Title X Clinics at a reduced rate. Family planning clinics with Title X funding can be searched here: https://www.opa-fpclinic db.com.

Long-Acting Reversible Contraception Counseling in Primary Care

With the knowledge that LARC methods are 20% more effective than CHCs, safe, recommended for use in nulliparous adolescents, and cost effective, the PCP should initiate contraceptive counseling by discussing LARC methods. Adolescents are often concerned about the process of placement; therefore, straightforward counseling with a focus on the long-term benefit and lack of regular maintenance can allay fears about discomfort with placement. Counseling always should include emphasis on the importance of vigilant condom use, given that there is no protection from STIs with contraceptive agents.

A qualitative study done at school-based health clinics in Washington State identified 5 factors that influence contraceptive choices by 14-year-old to 18-year-old girls in the primary care setting. Device-specific information, including effectiveness and lack of maintenance, is appealing to teenagers. Prior information from friends, family, and medical providers was important. Significant knowledge gaps were barriers to LARC use, which the PCPs can address. Teens were also motivated to use contraception for life circumstances, including avoiding pregnancy and going to college. Finally, environmental constraints and supports were found to be important, such as family expectations and the role of the PCP or school-based health center[23].

Dispelling common concerns

Adolescents gather information from many different places. Unfortunately, the information available about LARC methods can be out of date and misrepresented and there are many common misconceptions. Counseling that is attentive, honest, personalized, and confidential will dispel common myths and open a discussion of risks and benefits of LARC versus pregnancy (**Boxes 1** and **2; Table 5**).

Confidentiality

Laws protecting confidential access to contraception for minors vary by state. Many states allow mature minors to consent to reproductive care, including placement of LARCs. Updated information on confidentiality laws by state can be found at the Guttmacher Institute (guttmacher.org). Patients of all ages who are on their parents' insurance can have confidentiality broken when the explanation of benefits is sent home. There have been recent efforts to correct this, as many young adults now stay on their parents' insurance until they are 24 years old with the Affordable Care Act. However, the problem is complicated and multifaceted, balancing the need for transparency in cost with confidentiality for members, and it does not appear clear that a solution is

Box 1
Initial implant counseling

Placement	Done in a quick office procedure where one 4-cm flexible rod approximately the size of a matchstick is placed subdermally in the nondominant arm below the bicipital groove. The area is anesthetized with lidocaine, sterilized, and then the implant is placed by using a preloaded applicator. After placement, the area is kept bandaged for 3–5 days. Adolescents benefit from knowing that the procedure is quick and the only discomfort is when the lidocaine is placed.
Placement risks	Bleeding and infection at insertion site.
Menstrual bleeding	Regular menstrual cycles are interrupted. The ideal outcome ranges from light, painless menses to complete amenorrhea. It is not uncommon to have persistent irregular menstrual bleeding especially in the first 3 months.
Common reason for discontinuation	Implant users with persistent spotting after 3 to 4 months will likely continue with that pattern, and if the adolescent finds the bleeding pattern intolerable, additional management options, including removal, will be considered.

Box 2
Initial intrauterine device (IUD) counseling

Placement	An in-office procedure that requires the use of stirrups and speculum. Adolescent patients are counseled to take 600–800 mg ibuprofen before placement, because the procedure can be uncomfortable. The uterus is measured and then the IUD is placed through the cervix.
Placement risks	Discomfort, uterine perforation, infection, bleeding.
Levonorgestrel (LNG) IUD menstrual bleeding	Regular menstrual cycles are interrupted. The ideal outcome with LNG-containing IUDs ranges from light, painless menses to complete amenorrhea. It is not uncommon to have persistent irregular menstrual bleeding, especially in the first 3 months. With time, IUD users generally proceed to lighter menstrual bleeding.
Copper IUD menstrual bleeding	As previously stated, the bleeding outcomes from the copper IUD (Paraguard) is often heavy and therefore not commonly recommended for use in the adolescent population.

forthcoming. Therefore, if confidentiality absolutely cannot be broken, the adolescent patient should be sent to a Title X publicly funded clinic.

Finding a provider of long-acting reversible contraception

Providers who place LARC methods must be trained in these methods before placing them. Online resources for finding providers who place LARCs are available through the Association of Reproductive Health Professionals (larc.arhp.org) and bedsider. org. Most adolescent medicine clinics will have providers who place IUDs and implants. Adolescent patients also can be referred to local obstetrics/gynecology clinicians for placement. Planned Parenthood also places LARCs, which is important to consider, especially when confidentiality is a concern. If an appointment for LARC placement is not immediately available, it is wise for the PCP to consider the same-

Table 5
Dispelling common concerns about long-acting reversible contraception

Concern	Response
"My friend's intrauterine device (IUD) fell out"	Although it is possible to expel an IUD, it is very uncommon and can happen more often when an IUD is placed after pregnancy.
"I heard about someone who had an implant get lost (or broken)"	This is very uncommon and not likely. The rod is very flexible and not easily broken. Even if it does break, it is still effective. Removal of a broken implant might be more complicated. If you cannot feel the Nexplanon implant after placement, it can be located with a radiograph.
"My mom said IUDs are dangerous"	Prior generations of IUDs were found to have serious side effects, such as infection and infertility; however, those IUDs were completely taken off the market. The IUDs available now are widely used, well studied, and very safe.
"I can't use that because I have migraine headaches with aura"	Neither migraine with aura nor history of stroke, deep vein thrombosis, or pulmonary embolism are contraindications to use. LARC methods do not contain estrogen.
"Isn't the IUD used only for people who have had babies already?"	In past years, it was recommended that IUDs should be used only in women who had already given birth. That is no longer true today.
"Doesn't the IUD let fertilization happen but then stop the embryo from implanting in the uterus?"	No. Levonorgestrel IUDs prevent pregnancy by stopping ovulation, thickening the cervical mucus, making changes in the endometrium, and slowing motility of sperm.

day use of Depo-Provera injection in adolescents at high risk for pregnancy to buy time until placement can be scheduled.

After the long-acting reversible contraceptive is placed
Usually, adolescents are followed by the provider who placed the LARC if she has complaints or problems. On occasion, that individual will not be available, and the patient may turn to her PCP. In that case, clinicians should be aware of issues related to the management of those concerns (**Box 3**).

Challenges
A 2016 study published in *JAMA Pediatrics* on adolescent users of LARCs revealed an unsettling trend of lower condom use and greater numbers of sexual partners among adolescent LARC users versus sexually active adolescents using traditional birth control pills.[24] This puts adolescents using LARCs at higher risk of contracting STIs. PCPs will play an integral role in reversing this trend by counseling LARC users on the importance of condom use at each annual health care maintenance visit. When adolescents are not motivated to use condoms to prevent transmission of STIs, they can often be

---

Box 3
Management of common concerns

Irregular Bleeding

Irregular bleeding is the expected outcome of LARC methods, as the menstrual cycle is disrupted and ovulation is inhibited. However, with time, bleeding should become lighter, less painful, and infrequent. If irregular bleeding persists past the first few months, the adolescent should be referred back to the provider who placed the LARC for management of bleeding. After pregnancy and infection are ruled out, there are methods to manage undesirable bleeding.

Weight changes

Weight changes are possible, but are not an expected outcome of LARC. Patients presenting with weight concerns should be evaluated for more common lifestyle alterations, such as diet and exercise. Medical causes of weight changes also should be considered and ruled out before the LARC is considered the cause of weight gain or loss.

Acne

LARC methods do not have the secondary benefit of treating acne, as CHCs do. Adolescents with concerns about acne should be treated with traditional topical methods. However, adolescents who traditionally have acne flares with monthly menses will see a decrease in acne associated with menses, as monthly menses will likely be eliminated with LARC use.

Mood changes

Mood changes are not a frequent outcome of LARCs, and patients presenting with mood changes should be evaluated for more common causes of mood changes. However, mood changes can be attributed to hormones and any adolescent with persistent, unexplained, and undesirable mood changes should consider referral back to the LARC provider.

Return to fertility

Return to fertility is rapid after LARC removal. Adolescents who do not desire pregnancy should be counseled to use an alternate form of contraception as soon as the LARC is removed.

---

motivated by a gentle reminder that no method of contraception is 100% effective except for abstinence and that a condom is a must to prevent STIs and to prevent pregnancy.

SUMMARY

Long-acting reversible contraceptive devices are the ideal contraceptive options for sexually active adolescent girls. They are safe, effective, user friendly, well tolerated, and cost-effective. Adolescents stay on LARC methods longer than traditional contraceptive methods and rates of unintended pregnancy and abortion fall when they are used in the adolescent population. However, adolescents remain much more likely to be using less-effective methods, such as CHCs. Given their longitudinal relationship with teenagers and their parents, PCPs are the necessary catalyst to increasing the use of LARC among teenagers. With the information provided in this article, PCPs should feel more confident in recommending LARC methods to their adolescent patients.

REFERENCES

1. Committee on Adolescent Health Care Long-Acting Reversible Contraception Working Group, The American College of Obstetricians and Gynecologists. Committee opinion no. 539: adolescents and long-acting reversible contraception: implants and intrauterine devices. Obstet Gynecol 2012;120(4):983–8.
2. Committee on Adolescence. Contraception for adolescents. Pediatrics 2014; 134(4):e1244–56.
3. Abraham M, Zhao Q, Peipert JF. Young age, nulliparity, and continuation of long-acting reversible contraceptive methods. Obstet Gynecol 2015;126(4):823–9.
4. Diedrich JT, Zhao Q, Madden T, et al. Three-year continuation of reversible contraception. Am J Obstet Gynecol 2015;213(5):662.e1–8.
5. Rubin SE, Davis K, McKee MD. New York City physicians' views of providing long-acting reversible contraception to adolescents. Ann Fam Med 2013;11(2): 130–6.
6. National campaign to prevent teen and unplanned pregnancy. 2016. Available at: http://thenationalcampaign.org/data/landing. Accessed August 15, 2016.
7. Martinez GM, Abma JC. Sexual activity, contraceptive use, and childbearing of teenagers aged 15-19 in the United States. NCHS Data Brief 2015;(209):1–8.
8. CDC. Vital Signs: preventing teen pregnancy. 2015. Available at: http://www.cdc.gov/vitalsigns/larc/index.html. Accessed August 15, 2016.
9. Daniels K, Daugherty J, Jones J. Current contraceptive use and variation by selected characteristics among women aged 15-44: United States, 2011-2013. Natl Health Stat Report 2015;(86):1–14.
10. Nexplanon (etonogestrel-releasing device) [package insert]. Whitehouse Station, NJ: Merck & CO, INC; 2016.
11. Paragard T 380A (intrauterine copper contraceptive) [package insert]. Sellersville, PA: Teva Women's Health.
12. Skyla (levonorgestrel-releasing intrauterine system) [package insert]. Wayne, NJ: Bayer Healthcare Pharmaceuticals; 2013.
13. Mirena (levonorgestrel-releasing intrauterine system) [package insert]. Wayne, NJ: Bayer Healthcare Pharmaceuticals; 2013.
14. Liletta (levonorgestrel-releasing intrauterine system) [package insert]. Parsippany, NJ: Actavis and Medicines360; 2015.
15. Ricketts S, Klingler G, Schwalberg R. Game change in Colorado: widespread use of long-acting reversible contraceptives and rapid decline in births among young, low-income women. Perspect Sex Reprod Health 2014;46(3):125–32.
16. Effectiveness of Family Planning Methods. 2015. Available at: http://www.cdc.gov/reproductivehealth/unintendedpregnancy/pdf/contraceptive_methods_508.pdf. Accessed August 15, 2016.
17. Hov GG, Skjeldestad FE, Hilstad T. Use of IUD and subsequent fertility–follow-up after participation in a randomized clinical trial. Contraception 2007;75(2):88–92.
18. Tiovonen J, Luukkainen T, Allonen H. Protective effect of intrauterine release of levonorgestrel on pelvic infection: three years' comparative experience of levonorgestrel- and copper-releasing intrauterine devices. Obstet Gynecol 1991; 77(2):261–4.
19. Shokeir T, Amr M, Abdelshaheed M. The efficacy of Implanon for the treatment of chronic pelvic pain associated with pelvic congestion: 1-year randomized controlled pilot study. Arch Gynecol Obstet 2009;280(3):437–43.

20. Walch K, Unfried G, Huber J, et al. Implanon versus medroxyprogesterone acetate: effects on pain scores in patients with symptomatic endometriosis–a pilot study. Contraception 2009;79(1):29–34.
21. Dilbaz B, Ozdegirmenci O, Caliskan E, et al. Effect of etonogestrel implant on serum lipids, liver function tests and hemoglobin levels. Contraception 2010; 81(6):510–4.
22. Curtis KM, Tepper NK, Jatlaoui TC, et al. U.S. medical eligibility criteria for contraceptive use, 2016. MMWR Recomm Rep 2016;65(3):1–103.
23. Hoopes AJ, Gilmore K, Cady J, et al. A qualitative study of factors that influence contraceptive choice among adolescent school-based health center patients. J Pediatr Adolesc Gynecol 2016;29(3):259–64.
24. Steiner RJ, Liddon N, Swartzendruber AL, et al. Long-acting reversible contraception and condom use among female US high school students: implications for sexually transmitted infection prevention. JAMA Pediatr 2016;170(5):428–34.

Sometimes You Do Get a Second Chance

Emergency Contraception for Adolescents

Ellen S. Rome, MD, MPH[a,b],*, Veronica Issac, MD[a]

KEYWORDS

- Emergency contraception • Hormonal contraception • Unprotected intercourse
- Adolescents • Teen pregnancy • Pregnancy prevention

KEY POINTS

- Emergency contraception (EC) needs to be available, accessible, and proactively prescribed and/or discussed with adolescents before the need to use it.
- Counseling about EC does not result in increased sexual activity and can actively help prevent adolescent pregnancies.
- The copper T intrauterine device works very well and provides so-called forgettable contraception for up to 10 years after insertion.
- Ulipristal acetate is less expensive and has efficacy up to 5 days after intercourse, compared with levonorgestrel EC, with efficacy for up to 72 hours after unplanned intercourse.

INTRODUCTION

Emergency contraception (EC) is defined as any medication or device used to reduce the risk of pregnancy after unprotected or inadequately protected sexual intercourse. EC is intended as an emergency rescue measure in women who have had unprotected intercourse or a failure of another contraceptive method and is not intended to be used as a primary contraceptive method. In the United States, there are 4 currently approved methods of EC, including the copper intrauterine device (IUD) and 3 oral methods: ulipristal acetate (UPA), levonorgestrel, and the Yuzpe method (ethinyl

Conflicts of Interest: Dr E.S. Rome serves on the Merck Vaccine Advisory Board and Speakers Bureau. Dr V. Issac has no conflicts of interest.
No internal or external funding has been received for support of this article.
[a] Center for Adolescent Medicine, Cleveland Clinic Children's Hospital, A120, 9500 Euclid Avenue, Cleveland, OH 44195, USA; [b] Cleveland Clinic Lerner College of Medicine, Cleveland, OH, USA
* Corresponding author. Center for Adolescent Medicine, Cleveland Clinic Children's Hospital, A120, 9500 Euclid Avenue, Cleveland, OH 44195.
E-mail address: Romee@ccf.org

Pediatr Clin N Am 64 (2017) 371–380
http://dx.doi.org/10.1016/j.pcl.2016.11.006
0031-3955/17/© 2017 Elsevier Inc. All rights reserved.

estradiol plus levonorgestrel). Internationally, mifepristone is also approved in some countries for the purposes of EC. Compared with adults, adolescents are more likely to use contraception intermittently or ineffectively. In addition, adolescents are more likely than adults to use less effective forms of contraception.[1] Thus, sexually active adolescents are at high risk for unwanted or unplanned pregnancy compared with adults and are an important target for EC education and usage. Usage of EC in adolescents greatly improves if they receive counseling and prescriptions for usage before any need arises[2] **(Table 1)**.

EPIDEMIOLOGY

Despite decreases in the rate of teen births over the past 50 years in the United States, the teen birth rate remains high compared with other industrialized nations.[3,4] In addition, 82% of pregnancies in girls aged 15 to 19 years are unplanned or unintended.[5] Thus, adolescents represent an important target group for education not only about ongoing contraceptive options but also in the use of EC after unprotected intercourse, contraceptive failure, or sexual assault. The benefits of EC, in addition to preventing unintended pregnancy, also extend to related consequences of adolescent motherhood, including premature birth, stunted educational and vocational opportunities, decreased rates of high school completion, increased welfare dependence and future poverty rates, decreased psychological functioning, and decreased employment stability.[6]

PREGNANCY RISK

Ovulation usually occurs between days 10 and 21 of the menstrual cycle, most commonly between days 13 and 16. However, because adolescents are more likely to have irregular and/or anovulatory cycles, it is harder to predict when ovulation will occur. The fertile period is estimated to last about 6 days, beginning about 5 days before ovulation. Once an ovum is released, it has 24 hours to be fertilized by a spermatozoon. Spermatozoa remain viable in the female reproductive tract for 5 to 6 days and can fertilize an ovum on release from the ovaries during this time period.

Following a single act of intercourse at an unknown point in the menstrual cycle, there is a 4% to 6% risk of pregnancy.[7] However, during the most fertile time of the cycle (starting 5 days before ovulation and ending 24 hours after ovulation), this risk increases to approximately a 30% risk of becoming pregnant following a single encounter of vaginal intercourse.[7,8] Given the uncertainty of timing of ovulation, especially in adolescents, and the prolonged viability of sperm, EC should be encouraged in the setting of contraceptive failure at any point throughout the menstrual cycle. Adolescents suspected to require EC in the fertile window of the menstrual cycle may benefit from one of the more effective methods of EC, such as a copper IUD or UPA.

THE HISTORICAL (AND POLITICAL) PERSPECTIVE

The earliest EC in the Unites States used high-dose oral estrogen, which had side effects such as nausea and breast tenderness.[9,10] In the 1970s, the copper IUD as well as the Yuzpe method gained popularity; the latter consisted of a 2-dose regimen of 100 µg of ethinyl estradiol plus either 0.5 mg of levonorgestrel or 1.0 mg of norgestrel given 12 hours apart within 72 hours of sexual intercourse. The Yuzpe method was most commonly used in adolescents until the turn of the twenty-first century, when progestin-only methods were approved and became more popular; these

Table 1
Emergency contraception summary

Method (Trade Name)	Mechanism of Action	Benefits	Side Effects	Contraindications/ Considerations	Efficacy; Failure Rate (%)	Access	Cost ($)
Copper IUD (Paragard)	Prevents sperm motility to prevent fertilization	No hormone; can remain in place as contraception for 10 y	Heavier bleeding and/or cramping	Pregnancy, pelvic infection, allergy to copper	2.00	Must be placed by physician	500–932
UPA (Ella One)	Prevents or delays ovulation	Dose does not decline over time; 1-time dosing; side effects much less than estrogen-containing methods	Nausea and vomiting	Less effective in women with BMI>30 and ineffective in those with BMI>35, still more effective than levonorgestrel in this population	1.80	Requires prescription	33–36
Mifepristone (RU486)	Prevents or delays ovulation and affects endometrial development	Dose does not decline over time; 1-time dosing	Nausea and vomiting; cramping; bleeding	Abortifacient at high doses	2.19	Requires prescription; only available in certain countries	—
Levonorgestrel (Plan B, Plan B One-Step, Next Choice)	Prevents or delays ovulation	1-time dosing; side effects much less than estrogen-containing methods	Nausea and vomiting	Less effective with BMI>25 and ineffective for BMI>30 with failure rate of 5.8%	0.6–3.1	Available OTC	33–36
Ethinyl estradiol + levonorgestrel (Yuzpe method)	Prevents or delays ovulation	Widely available	Nausea and vomiting	Multiple doses with numerous pills; most side effects of all EC methods	—	Requires prescription	—

Abbreviations: BMI, body mass index; OTC, over the counter.

progestin-only methods had the advantages of less nausea (from no involving high-dose estrogen), easier dosing with 1-step administration, and reducing costs (UPA is currently half the price of Plan B One-Step in many American pharmacies). Moreover, pediatricians could prescribe progestins without the skill, training, time, and expertise required for IUD placement, which is a procedure that many gynecologists and, more recently, adolescent medicine specialists have been trained to perform for EC purposes.

In the United States, attitudes as well as policy with respect to EC access for adolescents has made progress forward and backward over the past several decades. In 1994, a survey of 167 adolescent health experts' attitudes on over-the-counter (OTC) EC revealed the following[11]:

- Twelve percent thought that providing OTC EC would encourage adolescent contraceptive risk taking
- Twenty-five percent thought that providing OTC EC would discourage correct use of other methods
- Twenty-nine percent thought that repeated use of EC would pose health risks to the adolescent
- Thirty-four percent stated that they would give out OTC EC provisions from their office
- Only 15% thought that EC should be available OTC[11]

Five years later, in 1999, levonorgestrel EC was approved by the US Food and Drug Administration (FDA) for prescription use for women more than 17 years of age. In 2002, California made a landmark decision to approve EC in the form of levonorgestrel emergency contraceptive pills for women of any age OTC through the state's pharmacy access laws. In 2003, the FDA's Advisory Committees for Reproductive Health Drugs and Nonprescription Drugs conducted an extensive review of the topic, resulting in the FDA recommending OTC Plan B (levonorgestrel, manufactured by Teva Women's Health, Woodcliff Lake, NJ) without any age restrictions.[12] However, the political debate continued to keep access limited, made more complicated by public confusion over all ECs being perceived as abortifacient.[10] Three years later, in 2006, OTC Plan B was legalized for girls aged 17 years and older, and only by prescription for girls younger than 17 years, ignoring the FDA's 2003 recommendation for approval of OTC Plan B for all ages. In 2011, the FDA recommendation was again ignored, when the Department of Health and Human Services only approved OTC sale of Plan B One-Step for youth 17 years and older.[12] In April 2013, OTC purchase of Plan B One-Step for boys (to buy for their female partners) and girls aged 15 years and older was legalized. By June 2013, those age restrictions were removed, allowing access to Plan B One-Step, with the explicit goal of decreasing the teen pregnancy rate.[10]

Health care organizations have also weighed in on this discussion. In 2012, the American Academy of Pediatrics (AAP) issued a policy statement recommending that pediatricians advocate for increased nonprescription access to EC for adolescents as well as for insurance coverage of EC to reduce cost barriers for adolescents.[13] Wilkinson and colleagues[14] performed mystery calls to nearly 1000 pharmacies across the United States; 759 pharmacies (80%) told adolescents and 766 (81%) told pediatricians that emergency contraceptive pill (ECP) was available OTC at their pharmacy; however, 45 (10%) of these pharmacies incorrectly told adolescents that they could not obtain ECP under any circumstances, and 23 (3%) of the pharmacies shared that same information with physicians.[14] Moreover, other barriers to care were directly observed, with adolescent mystery callers put on hold twice as often (54% vs 26%), with 36% of adolescents and 33% of adult mystery callers given no information on where to find OTC EC if it were unavailable at that pharmacy. In addition, only 5% of the pharmacies were open 24 hours a day, creating another barrier to care.[14]

SPECIFIC FORMS OF EMERGENCY CONTRACEPTION
Indications for and Timing of Emergency Contraceptive Use

Copper intrauterine device
Of the methods currently on the market, the copper IUD remains the most effective at preventing unintended pregnancy, with a pregnancy rate of 0.09%.[15] The copper IUD is the only nonhormonal method of EC. It is thought to work primarily by inhibiting sperm motility to prevent fertilization. To be most effective at preventing pregnancy, the IUD should be placed within 5 to 7 days of unprotected intercourse, but, as with other methods, earlier is better. Thus, in order to use it as EC, the device must be on hand and the patient must be able to obtain an appointment within the 5-day window with a skilled clinician trained in insertion. Once placed, this method can remain in place as so-called forgettable contraception for up to a decade, making it the only emergency contraceptive method with longevity of usage. Risks of use, including pelvic infection, expulsion, or perforation (1 in 1000), are low. The copper IUD is not affected by weight, making it an effective method of EC for obese girls and women. Levonorgestrel-containing IUDs (also called intrauterine systems) are not yet approved as ECs.

Marketed as: CuT-380A or Cu-375 SL IUD (ParaGuard).

Mechanism of action: prevents sperm motility to prevent fertilization.

Cost: as of July 2016 in several Ohio pharmacies, cost averaged $500 to $932, fully covered under most insurance plans.

Efficacy: 2% risk of pregnancy when given within 5 days of unplanned sexual activity.

Access: requires insertion in a skilled and trained physician's office or care setting.

Limitations: availability in pharmacy; access to skilled physician within 5 days of sexual activity; awareness as an option, with gaps in knowledge by clinicians, patients, and families.

Contraindications and side effects: side effects of copper IUD are caused by changes in the menstrual cycle, including heavier and/or prolonged bleeding and more cramping. This method is contraindicated in anyone who has an active pelvic infection, pregnancy, or allergy to copper (ie, Wilson disease).

Ulipristal acetate
UPA, a selective progesterone receptor modulator approved in the United States in June 2010, is considered the most effective hormonal method of EC. Used now in 79 countries, UPA has a pregnancy rate ranging from 0.9% to 2.1%.[16,17] UPA works by preventing or delaying ovulation when given before the onset of the luteinizing hormone (LH) surge, with additional efficacy after the onset of the LH surge but before the LH peak, with a direct inhibitory effect on follicular rupture.[16–18] Before the LH surge, it significantly delays follicular rupture; after the LH surge but before the LH peak it still has a direct inhibitory effect on follicular rupture.[17,18] Follicular rupture is delayed by 4 to 10 days, so a second method of protection is necessary until the next period.

The recommended dose for EC use is 30 mg given once orally. Given that ulipristal binds progesterone receptors, clinicians need to be mindful that it may interfere with progestin-containing contraceptives such as subdermal implants, depot medroxyprogesterone acetate, progestin-only contraceptives, and also combined oral contraceptives. As with all ECs, adolescents need to be reminded to use back-up protection, ideally all the time, but at a minimum until the next menstrual cycle.

It has been approved for use within 5 days of unprotected sexual intercourse, with equal efficacy over the entire 120-hour span; it is as effective on day 1 as on day 5. In contrast, the use of levonorgestrel EC on day 5 was associated with a 5-fold increased risk of pregnancy compared with levonorgestrel EC on day 1.[16]

A randomized controlled trial of levonorgestrel EC versus ulipristal given within 72 hours of unplanned sexual activity revealed pregnancy rates of 2.6% versus 1.8% respectively, with increased efficacy for ulipristal also at 120 hours.[16] UPA can be affected by a women's body mass index (BMI). It has been shown to be less effective in women with BMI greater than 30 and ineffective in those with BMI greater than 35, with a failure rate of 2.6%. However, its failure rate with obese women remains lower than levonorgestrel-containing EC.

Marketed as: Ella One

Dose: 30 mg given orally within 5 days of unplanned intercourse

Mechanism of action: prevents or delays ovulation as a selective progestin receptor modulator

Cost: as of July 2016 in several Ohio pharmacies, cost averaged $33 to $36

Efficacy: 1.8% risk of pregnancy when given within 5 days of unplanned sexual activity

Access: requires prescription (mystery call check)

Limitations: availability in pharmacy; gaps in knowledge by clinicians, patients, and families; less effective in women with BMI greater than 30 and with BMI greater than 35, failure rate 2.6%

Side effects: less nausea and vomiting than the traditional estrogen-containing Yuzpe method

Mifepristone

Mifepristone is an oral antiprogesterone. It is very effective as an EC, with similar pregnancy rates to ulipristal; in one study, mifepristone had a pregnancy rate of 1.48% given on days 1 to 3, and 2.19% given on days 4 to 5, compared with levonorgestrel 1.5 mg (1.34% at days 1–3, 2.67% at day4-5) and levonorgestrel 0.75 mg given as 2 doses (1.69% for days 1–3, 2.44% for days 4–5).[19] However, mifepristone, is only available for use as EC in a few countries. Mifepristone prevents or delays ovulation. It has also been shown to be effective after ovulation by affecting endometrial development. It must be given within 5 days of unprotected intercourse to be effective. Like UPA, its efficacy does not decline over time. Mifepristone can be given in an intermediate (25–50 mg) or low (<25 mg) dose as EC. At higher doses (600 mg), this medication serves as an abortifacient. It is important to discuss this distinction with patients when counseling about use as an emergency contraceptive method.

Marketed as: RU486

Mechanism of action: prevents or delays ovulation and affects endometrial development; low dose works as EC; high dose works as abortifacient

Efficacy: 2.19% risk of pregnancy when given within 5 days of unplanned sexual activity

Side effects: nausea and vomiting; cramping; bleeding

Access: not easily or legally obtainable in the United States (mystery call check).

Limitations: no availability in pharmacy, stigma associated with high-dose usage in the United States

Cost: not applicable in the United States

Levonorgestrel

Levonorgestrel, most commonly known as Plan B (2-dose version, 0.75 mg given orally 12 hours apart) and Plan B One-Step (1.5 mg), is probably the most widely known and most commonly used method of EC that is available worldwide. Although its pregnancy rate is higher than that of UPA or mifepristone, especially after 72 hours, it still is a highly effective method of EC, with rates ranging from 0.6% to 3.1%. It is most effective when given immediately after unplanned sexual activity. If given within 24 hours, 95% of pregnancies were prevented; from 25 to 48 hours, that rate decreases to 85%; and from 49 to 72 hours, the rate further decreases to 58%.[17,20] In contrast, the classic Yuzpe method of combined ethinyl estradiol and progestin resulted in pregnancies prevented in 77%, 36%, and 31% of patients respectively.[20] The 12-hour, 2-dosing 0.75-mg schedule was compared with the 1.5-mg single-dosing schedule in a multicenter World Health Organization (WHO) trial of more than 4000 women given EC within 120 hours of unplanned intercourse, with pregnancy rates of 1.8% versus 1.5% respectively.[19,20] Thus, ease of use of single dosing is justified and now normative in adolescents.

The mechanism of action involves prevention of follicular rupture and ovulation, but with little to no effect if the LH surge has begun or on postovulatory events.[17] Levonorgestrel is an oral progesterone that is given in a 1-time dose of 1.5 mg. It works by preventing or delaying ovulation only up to the LH surge. In a study of 99 women using levonorgestrel EC with the tracking of hormones to determine ovulation, those women given EC 2 to 5 days before ovulation had no pregnancies, whereas women given levonorgestrel EC on the day of or day after ovulation had the expected pregnancy rate.[21] Durand and colleagues[22] found that ovulatory women who took levonorgestrel EC had no changes in endometrial histology, but 80% of women taking EC on day 10 of the cycle were anovulatory.[22] Noé and colleagues[23] found zero pregnancies in the 87 women taking EC on days -5 to -1 before ovulation, with 13 pregnancies expected statistically, and 6 pregnancies in the 36 women taking EC on the day of ovulation or after, with 7 pregnancies expected. These studies confirm that levonorgestrel EC is not abortifacient but works to prevent follicular rupture and ovulation; because adolescents often are unclear on when they ovulate, ulipristal or copper T insertion remain more useful options when available.

Levonorgestrel is most effective when taken as soon as possible after unprotected intercourse but can be given up to 5 days (120 hours) after. Unlike both UPA and mifepristone, its efficacy does decline over time and therefore it might not be as effective if given further out. Furthermore, levonorgestrel is affected by body weight. This method becomes less effective with BMI greater than 25 and ineffective for BMI greater than 30, with a failure rate of 5.8%. Thus, UPA is a better option as oral EC for this population.

Marketed as: Plan B (0.75 mg for 2 doses given 12 hours apart), Plan B One-Step (1.5 mg), and Next Choice (two 0.75-mg tablets that can be taken at once)
Mechanism of action: prevents or delays ovulation
Cost: as of July 2016 in several Ohio pharmacies, cost averaged $33 to $36
Efficacy: 0.6% to 3.1% given within 3 days of unplanned sexual activity
Access: requires prescription (mystery call check); available OTC
Limitations: availability in pharmacy; gaps in knowledge by clinicians, patients, and families
Side effects: less nausea and vomiting than estrogen-containing EC (14%–23% vs 50% for nausea, 1%–6% vs 20% for vomiting)[17]; less effective with BMI greater than 25 and ineffective for BMI greater than 30, with failure rate of 5.8%

Yuzpe method (ethinyl estradiol + levonorgestrel)
The Yuzpe method is the least effective method with the most side effects. It is a combination of estrogen and progestin given orally in 2 doses divided 12 hours apart. Combined EC products are no longer available but can be formulated using a variety of oral contraceptive pills. Side effects include nausea and vomiting. It can be given within 5 days of unprotected intercourse. This method should not be considered first line for EC and should only be offered if no other method is available.

> Dosing: if the 50-μg ethinyl estradiol pill is available (Ovral), give 2 tablets orally every 12 hours for 2 doses. If the 30-μg to 35-μg ethinyl estradiol pills are available, give 4 pills every 12 hours for 2 doses. If only 20-μg ethinyl estradiol pills are available, the dose is 5 pills every 12 hours for 2 doses. With each of these formulations, an antiemetic should be given 30 minutes before each dose; some antiemetics, such as meclizine, may increase drowsiness.
> Timing: most effective within 72 hours of unplanned intercourse.
> Mechanism of action:
> Efficacy: similar to levonorgestrel EC.
> Access: currently requires prescription for adolescents and adults.

COMMON MYTHS AND MISCONCEPTIONS ABOUT EMERGENCY CONTRACEPTION

- EC does not affect implantation of a fertilized egg. These methods only work to inhibit pregnancy before fertilization (with the exception of mifepristone, which is the only EC that is also an abortifacient when given in high doses).
- Studies show that high-dose oral contraceptives do not pose any increased risk to an established pregnancy.[24] There is no teratogenicity with levonorgestrel EC, ulipristal EC, or the Yuzpe method.
- Talking about sex and prescribing or dispensing EC before it is needed does not make teens more sexually active. When clinicians have conversations about reproductive health over a lifespan and a healthy sexuality, including but not limited to the choice of abstinence, adolescents tend to reinforce their own healthy attitudes and behaviors and have less sexual activity than those receiving no counseling.
- Do not forget the boys. Since 2012, boys more than 18 years of age have been able legally to buy OTC EC. Talking about EC and dual methods of protection (optimally, long-acting reversible contraceptives [LARCs] for their partners plus condoms always until they are on their honeymoon) can help provide words and context for boys to make healthy choices about their sexuality.

A prescription or access to EC can begin a process of counseling that reinforces healthy choices designed to prevent unplanned pregnancy and prevent sexually transmitted infections. Because LARCs have now been recommended by the WHO (World Health Organization), AAP (American Academy of Pediatrics), Society for Adolescent Health and Medicine, American College of Obstetricians and Gynecologists, and US Centers for Disease Control and Prevention as first-line contraceptive choices for adolescents, the copper T IUD has some added benefits as a potential LARC, especially because it works well for a decade after insertion.[25,26] Any EC opportunity provides the chance to counsel adolescents using motivational interviewing to ensure the use of dual methods of contraception for those youth engaged in heterosexual sexual activity, and condom use for all youth engaging in sexual activity of all forms.

ACKNOWLEDGMENTS

The authors acknowledge with gratitude the efforts of Erin Sieke, medical student at the Cleveland Clinic Lerner College of Medicine, for her assistance with this article and for her articulate thought processes in all aspects of adolescent medicine. Medical students were not permitted to be coauthors for this edition; we wish the honor could be shared with her, and we eagerly look forward to all of her future contributions as she continues to pursue excellence in adolescent medicine.

REFERENCES

1. Harper CC, Cheong M, Rocca CH, et al. The effect of increased access to emergency contraception among young adolescents. Obstet Gynecol 2005;106: 483–91.
2. Meyer JL, Gold MA, Haggerty CL. Advance provision of emergency contraception among adolescent and young adult women: a systematic review of literature. J Pediatr Adolesc Gynecol 2011;24:2–9.
3. Ventura SJ, Curtin SC, Abma JC, et al. Estimated pregnancy rates and rates of pregnancy outcomes for the United States, 1990-2008. Natl Vital Stat Rep 2012;60:1–21.
4. Martinez G, Copen CE, Abma JC. Teenagers in the United States: sexual activity, contraceptive use, and childbearing, 2006-2010 national survey of family growth. Vital Health Stat 23 2011;(31):1–35.
5. Finer LB, Zolna MR. Unintended pregnancy in the United States: incidence and disparities, 2006. Contraception 2011;84:478–85.
6. Molina Cartes R, González Araya E. Teenage pregnancy. Endocr Dev 2012;22: 302–31.
7. Wilcox AJ, Dunson DB, Weinberg CR, et al. Likelihood of conception with a single act of intercourse: providing benchmark rates for assessment of post-coital contraceptives. Contraception 2001;63:211–5.
8. Glasier A, Cameron ST, Blithe D, et al. Can we identify women at risk of pregnancy despite using emergency contraception? Data from randomized trials of ulipristal acetate and levonorgestrel. Contraception 2011;84:363–7.
9. Ellertson C. History and efficacy of emergency contraception: beyond Coca-Cola. Fam Plann Perspect 1996;28:44–8.
10. Society for Adolescent Health and Medicine. Emergency contraception for adolescents and young adults: guidance for health care professionals. J Adolesc Health 2016;58:245–8.
11. Gold MA, Schein A, Coupey SM. Emergency contraception: a national survey of adolescent health experts. Fam Plann Perspect 1997;29:15–9, 24.
12. Wood AJJ, Drazen JM, Greene MF. The politics of emergency contraception. N Engl J Med 2012;366:101–2.
13. Committee On Adolescence. Emergency contraception. Pediatrics 2012. http://dx.doi.org/10.1542/peds.2012-2962.
14. Wilkinson TA, Fahey N, Shields C, et al. Pharmacy communication to adolescents and their physicians regarding access to emergency contraception. Pediatrics 2012;129;624–9.
15. Cleland K, Zhu H, Goldstuck N, et al. The efficacy of intrauterine devices for emergency contraception: a systematic review of 35 years of experience. Hum Reprod 2012;27:1994–2000.

16. Glasier AF, Cameron ST, Fine PM, et al. Ulipristal acetate versus levonorgestrel for emergency contraception: a randomised non-inferiority trial and meta-analysis. Lancet 2010;375:555–62.
17. Emans SJ, Laufer MR. Pediatric and Adolescent Gynecology. 6th edition. Lippincott Williams & Wilkins; 2011.
18. Brache V, Cochon L, Jesam C, et al. Immediate pre-ovulatory administration of 30 mg ulipristal acetate significantly delays follicular rupture. Hum Reprod 2010;25:2256–63.
19. von Hertzen H, Piaggio G, Ding J, et al. Low dose mifepristone and two regimens of levonorgestrel for emergency contraception: a WHO multicentre randomised trial. Lancet 2002;360:1803–10.
20. von Hertzen H, Piaggio G. Emergency contraception with levonorgestrel or the Yuzpe regimen. Lancet 1998;352:1939.
21. Novikova N, Weisberg E, Stanczyk FZ, et al. Effectiveness of levonorgestrel emergency contraception given before or after ovulation–a pilot study. Contraception 2007;75:112–8.
22. Durand M, del Carmen Cravioto M, Raymond EG, et al. On the mechanisms of action of short-term levonorgestrel administration in emergency contraception. Contraception 2001;64:227–34.
23. Noé G, Croxatto HB, Salvatierra AM, et al. Contraceptive efficacy of emergency contraception with levonorgestrel given before or after ovulation. Contraception 2010;81:414–20.
24. Practice bulletin summary no. 152: emergency contraception. Obstet Gynecol 2015;126:685–6.
25. Curtis KM, Tepper NK, Jatlaoui TC, et al. U.S. medical eligibility criteria for contraceptive use, 2016. MMWR Recomm Rep 2016;65:1–103.
26. World Health Organization, Reproductive Health and Research & World Health Organization. Medical eligibility criteria for contraceptive use. 2015.

Adolescent Pregnancy

Heidi K. Leftwich, DO[a],*, Marcus Vinicius Ortega Alves, MD[b]

KEYWORDS

- Adolescent pregnancy • Teen pregnancy • Unintended pregnancy

KEY POINTS

- Adolescent pregnancy is a significant public health concern, occurring in approximately 13% of the United States population and approximately 25% of women worldwide.
- Adolescent mothers are at high risk for rapid repeat pregnancy in the 1 to 2 years after their initial pregnancy.
- Long-acting reversible contraception decreases the rates of rapid repeat pregnancy in the adolescent population and should be offered to those wanting long-term pregnancy prevention.

OVERVIEW

Adolescent pregnancy, typically defined as a pregnancy in a female between the ages of 13 and 19, occurs in approximately 13% of the United States population and approximately 25% of women worldwide.[1,2] Although high, this rate has been steadily declining over the last 15 years,[3] owing to support of education, contraception, and other pregnancy prevention strategies. When looking at teens between 15 and 19 years of age, the birth rate was 24.2 per 1000 in 2014, down 9% from 2013.[3] Even with the decrease, in 2008, approximately 7% of teenage girls in the United States became pregnant.[4] Approximately 80% of pregnancies conceived during adolescence are unintended. Teen births are highest in those cohabiting, married, and in lower income groups.[5] Those aged 18 to 19 years make up the vast majority of teen pregnancies, between 64% and 76%.[6] This high rate of unintended pregnancy correlates to a high rate of abortions in this population, with 1 study reporting that up to 50% of teen pregnancies lead to abortions.[7] Not only specific to the United States, adolescent pregnancy is a global health problem, with complications during pregnancy and childbirth serving as the second leading cause of mortality in the 15- to 19-year-old age group worldwide.[8] In the United States, preventing unintended

Disclosure: The authors have nothing to disclose.
[a] Division of Maternal-Fetal Medicine, Department of Obstetrics and Gynecology, University of Massachusetts Medical School, 119 Belmont Street, Worcester, MA 01605, USA; [b] Department of Obstetrics and Gynecology, University of Massachusetts Medical School, 119 Belmont Street, Worcester, MA 01605, USA
* Corresponding author.
E-mail address: heidi.leftwich@umassmemorial.org

http://dx.doi.org/10.1016/j.pcl.2016.11.007

adolescent pregnancies is part of the Healthy People 2020 campaign. Promoting safe sex and having access to contraception for these individuals continues to be part of this objective.[4]

Adolescent pregnancy contributes highly to the financial, emotional, and social well-being of the pregnant teen.[1,9] Many of these factors are compounded by the fact that teenagers have greater risk of poor nutrition, delayed pregnancy diagnosis, and delayed access to prenatal care. They are often plagued by poor social support and emotional well-being, compared with adult women. Pregnant teens have higher use of tobacco (36% vs 7%) and alcohol and recreational drugs (1.1% vs 0.2%), as well as higher levels of emotional stress, partner violence and abandonment, and unstable and/or unsafe home environments.[1,4,8] Having a child while in school significantly decreases the chance of completion of high school, with as many as 30,000 citing pregnancy or childbirth as reasons of dropout each year.[10] However, those pregnant adolescents who remain in school after childbirth are less likely to have a short-interval repeat pregnancy, making continued encouragement of the adolescent to complete her schooling even more important.[10] Pediatricians and other primary care providers can have such an important role in this counseling, especially before pregnancy diagnosis.[11] Additionally, pediatricians care for many potential teenage fathers and thus can also impact adolescent pregnancy rates through counseling regarding safe sex practices to all youth. By their 19th birthday, 7 of 10 teens in the United States have had sexual intercourse.[12]

Adolescent well visits are a perfect time to discuss delaying parenthood until after adolescence.[11] Contraceptive counseling and safe sex practices, when addressed in the pediatric or family practice office, can be a tool to help the adolescent make healthy decisions regarding their reproductive desires. Many adolescents feel immune to the possibility of pregnancy and therefore do not consider contraception until a health care provider initiates the discussion.[11] Social stressors of adolescent pregnancy should be addressed immediately with a collaborative, nonjudgmental environment of support through social work, and community resources, including Planned Parenthood, psychiatry if appropriate, as well as any local advocacy groups.

EARLY DIAGNOSIS OF PREGNANCY

Because early detection and therefore early referral of a pregnant adolescent can help to decrease perinatal risks,[9] it is imperative to not miss a diagnosis of pregnancy in an adolescent who presents to the office for vague complaints. Although some teens may present with more classic symptoms of amenorrhea, nausea, vomiting, breast tenderness, and/or weight gain, others may be more subtle, with complaints of fatigue, abdominal pain, dizziness, or overall "not feeling well."[4] Additionally, the menstrual cycle of an adolescent is often irregular and may give a false reassurance that a pregnancy does not need to be considered, thus causing a delay in diagnosis and prenatal care. Teens often feel they are not at risk for pregnancy, regardless of unprotected intercourse. Denial often plays a role in the patient's late presentation for medical care and ultimate diagnosis of pregnancy. However, this is why it is important to check a pregnancy test with menstrual irregularities, regardless of reported sexual history, because some patients are not forthcoming with regard to their sexual history. Alternatively, some adolescents will present to their pediatrician or family medicine physician with vague complaints, already knowing they are pregnant, to establish medical care.[4] Urine qualitative human chorionic gonadotropin tests are the gold standard for initial evaluation and may be repeated if negative in 1 to 2 weeks if suspicion is high.[4] Adolescent mothers are at greater risk for late or no prenatal care, with 9.1% of adolescents aged 15 to 16 years and 15.8% of those 10 to 14 years in 2003 having either no prenatal care or care starting after the second trimester.[13] In general, it is wise to consider the diagnosis of pregnancy frequently in the adolescent population.

ADVERSE PERINATAL OUTCOMES

Several adverse perinatal outcomes have been associated with adolescent pregnancies, specifically, preeclampsia, preterm birth, low birth weight babies, and an increase in stillbirths, intrapartum deaths, and miscarriages.[14,15] One study reports more than 4 times the risk of intrapartum stillbirth in the youngest teens (<15 years old) and 50% higher in teens 15 to 19 years old compared with women aged 20 to 24.[15] The highest risk of poor perinatal outcomes occurs in pregnancies taking place within 2 years of menarche.[16] A higher incidence of intrapartum stillbirth in this group has been postulated to be owing to increase in shoulder dystocia or intrapartum asphyxia owing to the immaturity of the young teenage body and bony pelvic structures, but this direct correlation has not been made.[15] Additionally, the younger the patient, the greater the risk, with rates of infant mortality, very low birth weight and preterm delivery significantly greater if pregnancy is diagnosed before 15 years old compared with older teens.[16] Lack of early prenatal care has been cited as one of the leading contributors to this problem, though not the only cause of these adverse outcomes in this patient population, and therefore serves as a focus of much research as to how to improve the outcomes in this high risk population.[9] Fraser and colleagues,[14] while studying a mainly homogenous population in Utah, demonstrated that younger maternal age was an independent risk factor for adverse pregnancy outcomes of important confounding sociodemographic factors, although did still note that inadequate prenatal care was mostly strongly correlating to adverse perinatal outcomes. Interestingly, although there are concerns with incomplete growth and biologic immaturity of the adolescent causing some of these poor outcomes, there is a decrease in the cesarean delivery rate in this population, suggesting that pelvic structure may in fact be sufficiently developed in most adolescents.[16] Preventable risks include late prenatal care initiation, poor nutrition, substance abuse and genital infections.[9,17] Primary care physicians who diagnose pregnancy in adolescent patients can be of great assistance in preventing poor outcomes and optimizing care for the mother and fetus.

ACTIONS THAT CAN BE TAKEN IN THE PEDIATRIC OFFICE

Obtaining and complying with adequate prenatal care, even when an early diagnosis of pregnancy is made, is often a challenge given the poor health behaviors of many adolescents and perceived limited prenatal care access. It is important to promote a safe, confidential avenue for patients to share their concerns regarding potential pregnancies to establish early diagnosis.[4] Pediatric providers must become comfortable talking about sexual issues for this to happen (See Betsy Pfeffer and colleagues' article, "Interviewing Adolescents about Sexual Matters," in this issue). Many adolescents will not share information regarding their sexual history unless specifically asked and if confidentiality is assured.[4] Early confirmation of dating by ultrasound examination is equally important, especially given the sometimes erratic nature of adolescent menstruation.[4] If unavailable in the office of the provider diagnosing the pregnancy, this should be ordered as soon as possible after diagnosis, if gestation is suspected to be greater than 6 weeks. Every effort should be made to help pregnant adolescents to initiate early prenatal care and adopt a healthy lifestyle. Even in late to care circumstances, early referral to an obstetric service will help to confirm dating and help to decrease the rates of poor perinatal outcomes. Girls who reach menarche before age 11 are considered very early maturers and are at increased risk for ectopic pregnancy.[16,18] Lack of diagnosis of ectopic pregnancy if present could end in significant hemorrhage from a ruptured ectopic and result in death, if untreated.

Options counseling should begin as soon as a positive pregnancy test is found. Pregnant teens should know that they have 3 options to consider: (1) continuing the pregnancy and parenting the child, (2) continuing the pregnancy and pursuing an adoption; and (3) terminating the pregnancy. Open-ended questions are the best way to discuss these with an adolescent patient.[4] Sample questions include:

Have you considered the fact that you could be pregnant?
Who do you trust to inform of this information?
Do you have adequate support at home?
Do you feel safe at home?
Is this pregnancy a result of consensual relations?
If so, is this person still in your life?
Will that person remain involved?
How old is the father of the baby?
What do you think will happen when you tell your parents you are pregnant?
Would you like assistance in telling your parents? (Here the clinician can assess for signs and symptoms of depression and ensure that the teenager does not have suicidal or homicidal ideation and that the patient is safe to go home.)

After these open-ended questions are reviewed, the clinician can have an open discussion with the adolescent patient regarding her decision of continuing the pregnancy and parenting the child, continuing the pregnancy and pursuing adoption services or electing not to continue the pregnancy and opting for termination.[4]

A specific focus on adequate nutrition, including supplementation of folic acid of 400 μg daily, should be discussed. Sexual health and practices during pregnancy should be addressed. Sexually transmitted infections are more prevalent in the adolescent population (See Zoon Wangu and Gale R. Burstein's article, "Adolescent Sexuality: Updates to the Sexually Transmitted Infection Guidelines," in this issue). Untreated sexually transmitted infections can have an increase in adverse perinatal outcomes.[8] Pregnant adolescents are more than 4 times more likely to have unprotected intercourse than nonpregnant teens.[19] Condom use is decreased even more in the third trimester, making this a high-risk time for infection.[19] Screening for sexually transmitted infections should, therefore, be more frequent and occur at the first prenatal visit, with diagnosis of pregnancy, as well as in the third trimester and with any complaint of abnormal vaginal discharge or a new partner.[8] Anemia is also very common in this population and it is found in about 50% of pregnant teens.[17] It is important to diagnose and treat underlying iron deficiency anemia to optimize the patient's health, well-being, and risk profile during the pregnancy and prepare for a delivery with fewer complications from anemia. Therefore, before referral to an obstetrician or midwife, it would be important to start prenatal vitamins and iron, if appropriate, upon diagnosis.

Depression is common in pregnant teens. In addition to depressive symptoms, social anxiety, limited support, poor self-esteem and increased stress plague this already vulnerable population.[11] Forty percent of adolescent mothers report feeling stigmatized by their pregnancy.[8] Approximately one-half of all adolescent mothers experience moderate to severe depression in the first postpartum year.[8] This puts a significant ownership on providers caring for this population to continually screen and offer support to help mitigate this risk. Another risk factor for adolescent pregnancy and subsequent poor perinatal outcomes is a history of adverse childhood experiences, including but not limited to emotional, physical, or sexual abuse; living with someone who suffers from substance abuse, mental illness, or has a criminal record; or having parents who are separated or divorced.[20] These risks must be assessed in the adolescent male population as well, because young men with such a history are more likely to father a child with an adolescent mother.[20] Male influence on intention of pregnancy may also have an impact on an adolescent girl's desiring pregnancy.[21] Therefore, efforts to prevent adolescent pregnancy should also start with discussion regarding a male partner's desire for a pregnancy.[20] Violence and coercion unfortunately continue to be a major problem for this population and seem to be quite common[20] (See Elizabeth Miller's article, "Prevention of and Interventions for Dating and Sexual Violence in Adolescence," in this issue). Intimate partner violence is common against pregnant women.[20] Lack of social support and high-risk behaviors contribute to the issue. Community-based programs can offer appropriate screening and help identified victims to find a safer and protected environment during this vulnerable time. Ideally, assessments for adverse childhood experiences should take place before adolescence to initiate support before the onset of high-risk behaviors leading to adolescent pregnancy. It is always important to screen for intimate partner violence. Not all adolescents who experience adverse childhood experiences exhibit high-risk behaviors. Having positive interactions such as feelings of self-worth and achievement, good parenting or at least mentorship, strong connection to extended family, and school and community can help these patients in breaking the cycle of high-risk behaviors.[20]

Standard prenatal care in most obstetric settings that care for adult women do not focus on psychological vulnerabilities, sexually transmitted infection screening, and postpartum issues such as breastfeeding, contraception, and school return. In addition, standard prenatal care might not be appropriate if additional nutrition and social work visits are necessary. Some special circumstances in the teenager's life might influence adherence to prenatal care such as school, transportation, or child care for their other children.[22,23] Additionally, the use of public health nursing care for post birth assistance helped to decreased the days of infant hospitalization and improved immunization rates in at least one study.[10] It seems that a multidisciplinary approach to the care of a pregnant adolescent can help to attain better compliance to prenatal care and thus improved outcomes for both mother and child.[10,17,21]

REPEAT PREGNANCY

Adolescent mothers have high rates of repeat pregnancy: 25% become pregnant again within 1 year of delivery and 35% within 2 years.[12] In fact, 20% of the births to adolescents in the United States are from repeat births.[12] Although this may be partially owing to noncompliance with a post partum visit, studies suggest that teenagers are less likely overall to be compliant with contraceptive methods, especially condoms and oral contraception, despite oral contraception being the preferred method with this patient population.[7] Failure rates of oral contraception are evident when rates of stated contraception use at time of conception for adolescents can vary between 36% and 80%.[7] In fact, in 2006, adolescents between the ages of 15 and 19 reported an 86% use of some method of contraception during their last sexual intercourse.[24] The discord in use and unintended pregnancy may be owing to limited knowledge of usage and failure rates, which shows that counseling regarding these options has the ability to improve usage and, therefore, could impact the rates of unintended pregnancies.

Teenagers who have a second pregnancy in their adolescent years have increase in poor perinatal outcomes, specifically extreme prematurity and stillbirth, than in their first adolescent pregnancy.[25] Approximately two-thirds of repeat pregnancies in this adolescent age group are reported as unintended and approximately one-half end in abortion, often in the second trimester owing to late diagnosis.[12] Clearly, the best method of contraception for sexually active adolescents is the safest, most effective method that they will continue to use. Therefore, counseling regarding cultural barriers, side effects, appropriate use, and failure rates may help patients to initially select the method that is right for them, which would improve adherence and prevent early discontinuation (See Anne Powell's article, "Choosing the Right Oral Contraceptive Pill for Teens," in this issue). Similarly, careful attention to the benefit of condom use to prevent sexually transmitted infections cannot be forgotten when discussing contraception.[12] Approximately 11% of women aged 16 to 19 diagnosed with a sexually transmitted infection in 2009 became reinfected within 1 year.[26,27] Early childhood interventions have been shown to be beneficial in reducing unintended pregnancies as well, and should be encouraged, reporting a 39% decrease in teenage pregnancy rate in those who participated in such interventions through social support, work experience, and career development.[8]

PREVENTION

After giving birth or having an abortion, many young women express a desire to avoid a pregnancy in the near future.[12] However, they often change their minds or become ambivalent over several months and have limited if any contraceptive method use or safe sex practices.[12] Adolescent mothers who had intended pregnancies, live with a male partner, had a preterm delivery, and/or resume sexual intercourse promptly after delivery are less likely to use contraception.[12] The fecundity rate is so high in this population that they have an approximately 90% chance of becoming pregnant within 1 year of unprotected intercourse.[12] Long-acting reversible contraception (LARC) via either intrauterine device or contraception implant can be an effective way to help prevent unintended rapid repeat pregnancies in this population.[12] LARC is now recommended by the American Academy of Pediatrics and the College of Obstetrics and Gynecology as the first line of contraception for adolescents overall. In general, LARC has a typical use effectiveness rate of greater than 99% and continuation usage after 1 year of 80% to 90% (See Suzanne Allen and Erin Barlow's article, "Long Acting Reversible Contraception: An essential guide for pediatric primary care providers," in this issue). When used at the time of initial abortion, LARC has been shown to decrease abortion rates. Women who received a LARC at the time of an abortion were less likely to have a repeat abortion compared with those who did not receive LARC (18.3 in 1000 vs 37.3 in 1000; $P<.01$).

Therefore, if an adolescent patient presents to a primary care office desiring contraception, it is important to include the option of LARC, even if a consult with a gynecologist would be appropriate for its eventual placement. Additionally, LARC methods in adolescents are effective in decreasing repeat pregnancy within 2 years, even when discontinued early, because the LARC for even a short period decreases the risk over the time that it was used.[12]

SUMMARY

Adolescent pregnancy, although on the decline, remains a significant public health concern. Often adolescents present late to prenatal care, either from lack of knowledge, fear of consequences, limited access, stigma, or all of these reasons. Although multifaceted, there are risks to both mother and child that are increased in adolescent pregnancy. Many adolescent pregnancies are unintended and those having unintended pregnancies are at risk for repeat adolescent pregnancy, especially in the 2 years after the first pregnancy. Risks include but are not limited to low birth weight, preterm delivery, stillbirth, and preeclampsia, as well as feelings of social isolation, delayed or neglected educational goals, and depression for the mother. Many of these risks can be minimized with multidisciplinary, prenatal care through early and nonjudgmental detection of pregnancy. Contraception, with specific attention to LARC, should be considered in this high-risk population to help prevent unintended first and repeat pregnancies.

REFERENCES

1. Chandra PC, Schiavello HJ, Ravi B, et al. Pregnancy outcomes in urban teenagers. Int J Gynaecol Obstet 2002;79:117–22.
2. Stewart CP, Katz J, Khatry SK, et al. Preterm delivery but not intrauterine growth restriction is associated with young maternal age among primiparae in rural Nepal. Matern Child Nutr 2007;3(3):174–85.
3. Hamilton BE, Martin JA, Osterman MJK, et al. Births: final data for 2014. Natl Vital Stat Rep 2015;64(12):1–64.
4. Dalby J, Hayon R, Carlson J. Adolescent pregnancy and contraception. Prim Care 2014;41(3):607–29.
5. Finer LB, Zolna MR. Unintended pregnancy in the United States: incidence and disparities, 2006. Contraception 2011;84(5):478–85.
6. Kost K, Henshaw S. U.S. teenage pregnancies, births and abortions, 2008; state trends by age, race and ethnicity. New York: Guttmacher Institute; 2013.
7. Falk G, Ostlund I, Magnuson A, et al. Teenage mothers—a high risk group for new unintended pregnancies. Contraception 2006;74:471–5.
8. McCarthy FP, O'Brien U, Kenny LC. The management of teenage pregnancy. BMJ 2014;349:g5887.
9. Mollborn S, Morningstar E. Investigating the relationship between teenage childbearing and psychological distress using longitudinal evidence. J Health Soc Behav 2009;50(3):310–26.
10. Koniak-Griffin D, Anderson NLR, Crecht ML, et al. Public health nursing care for adolescent mothers: impact on infant health and selected maternal outcomes at 1 year postbirth. J Adolesc Health 2002;30:44–54.
11. Block RW, Saltzman S, Block SA. Teenage pregnancy. Adv Pediatr 1981;28: 75–98.
12. Baldwin MK, Edelman AB. The effect of long-acting reversible contraception on rapid repeat pregnancy in adolescents: a review. J Adolesc Health 2013;52: S47–53.
13. Hueston WJ, Geesey MF, Diaz V. Prenatal care initiation among pregnant teens in the united states: an analysis over 25 years. J Adolesc Health 2008;42:243–8.
14. Fraser AM, Brockert JE, Ward RH. Association of young maternal age with adverse reproductive outcomes. N Engl J Med 1995;332(17):1113–7.
15. Wilson RE, Alio AP, Kirby RS, et al. Young maternal age and risk of intrapartum stillbirth. Arch Gynecol Obstet 2008;278:231–6.
16. Kramer KL, Lancaster JB. Teen motherhood in cross-cultural perspective. Ann Hum Biol 2010;37(5):613–28.
17. Soares NN, Mattar R, Camano L, et al. Iron deficiency anemia and iron stores in adult and adolescent women in pregnancy. Acta Obstet Gynecol Scand 2010;89: 343–9.

18. Sandler DP, Wilcox AJ, Horney LF. Age at menarche and subsequent reproductive events. Am J Epidemiol 1984;119(5):765–74.
19. Niccolai LM, Ethier KA, Kershaw TS, et al. Pregnant adolescents at risk: sexual behaviors and sexually transmitted disease prevalence. Am J Obstet Gynecol 2003;188:63–70.
20. Magill MK, Wilcox RW. Adolescent pregnancy and associated risks: not just a result of maternal age. Am Fam Physician 2007;75(9):1310–1.
21. Clear ER, Williams CM, Crosby RA. Female perceptions of male versus female intendedness at the time of teenage pregnancy. Matern Child Health J 2012; 16:1862–9.
22. Lao TT, Suen SS, Sahota DS, et al. Has improved health care provision impacted on the obstetric outcome in teenage women? J Matern Fetal Neonatal Med 2012; 25:1358–62.
23. Lao TT, Ho LF. Obstetric outcome of teenage pregnancies. Hum Reprod 1998;13: 3228–32.
24. Martinez G, Copen CE, Abma JC. Teenagers in the United States: sexual activity, contraceptive use, and childbearing, 2006-2010 National Survey of Family Growth. Series 23, data from the National Survey of Family Growth. Vital Health Stat 23 2011;(31):1–35.
25. Smith G, Pell JP. Teenage pregnancy and risk of adverse perinatal outcomes associated with first and second births: population based retrospective cohort study. BMJ 2001;323:476–9.
26. Hughes G, Field N. The epidemiology of sexually transmitted infections in the UK: impact of behavior, services and interventions. Future Microbiol 2015;10(1): 35–51.
27. Mestad R, Secura G, Allsworth JE, et al. Acceptance of long-acting reversible contraceptive methods by adolescent participants in the Contraceptive CHOICE project. Contraception 2011;84:493–8.

Adolescent Sexuality

Updates to the Sexually Transmitted Infection Guidelines

Zoon Wangu, MD[a,b,*], Gale R. Burstein, MD, MPH[c,d,e]

KEYWORDS

- Adolescents • Sexual health • Sexually transmitted infections
- Sexually transmitted diseases • Risk behaviors • Screening • Prevention

KEY POINTS

- Adolescents constitute one of the groups at highest risk for the acquisition and transmission of sexually transmitted infections (STI).
- Adolescents are both biologically and cognitively susceptible to acquisition of STIs.
- New guidelines are available regarding updates to the prevention, screening, diagnosis, and management of STIs in this age group.

INTRODUCTION

The Centers for Disease Control and Prevention (CDC) estimates that among the 20 million new sexually transmitted infections (STIs) diagnosed every year in the United States, one-half of these occur in young people aged 15 to 24 years.[1] Adolescents and young adults account for 53% of US reported gonorrhea cases and 65% of reported chlamydia cases.[1] Of concern, there has been an alarming increase in syphilis rates (15.1% from 2013 to 2014) among men who have sex with men (MSM), particularly those who are young and of color.

Adolescents are in a unique period of development; their psychosocial developmental stage is associated with increased risk-taking behaviors and desire for autonomy.[2] Their STI risk is multifactorial, including increased likelihood of multiple sex partners, lower levels of condom use, unprotected sex, complex structure of sexual

Disclosure of Potential Conflicts of Interest: No potential conflicts of interest were disclosed.
[a] Division of Pediatric Infectious Diseases & Immunology, UMass Memorial Children's Medical Center, 55 Lake Avenue North, Worcester, MA 01655, USA; [b] Ratelle STD/HIV Prevention Training Center, Massachusetts Department of Public Health, 305 South Street Stables Fl 2, Jamaica Plain, MA 02130, USA; [c] Division of Adolescent Medicine, SUNY at Buffalo School of Medicine and Biomedical Sciences, 131 Biomedical Education Building, Buffalo, NY 14260, USA; [d] Erie County Department of Health, 95 Franklin St, Buffalo, NY 14202, USA; [e] New York City STD/HIV Prevention Training Center, 125 Worth St, New York, NY 10013, USA
* Correspondence author.
E-mail address: zoon.wangu@umassmemorial.org

pediatric.theclinics.com

networks, adolescent female susceptibility to infection owing to cervical ectopy, older sexual partners, mental health issues and substance abuse, and less access to confidential STI prevention and clinical services.[1,3–6]

This article discusses the most common STIs encountered in adolescents, with an emphasis on new guidelines for diagnosis, treatment, and prevention.

CHLAMYDIA TRACHOMATIS INFECTIONS
Clinical Manifestations

Chlamydia is the most frequently reported infectious disease in the United States and is the second most common STI in US adolescents after human papillomavirus (HPV).[1] Although most infections are asymptomatic, clinical manifestations include urethritis, epididymitis, cervicitis, proctitis, pelvic inflammatory disease (PID), and conjunctivitis and pneumonia among infants. Chlamydia is one of the leading causes of tubal factor infertility in females, which is preventable with early detection and treatment. Although the clinical significance of oropharyngeal infection is unclear, available evidence suggests that C trachomatis can be sexually transmitted from oral to genital sites.[7]

Diagnosis and Screening

Nucleic acid amplification tests (NAATs) have superior sensitivity and adequate specificity compared with older nonculture and non-NAAT methods for the diagnosis of C trachomatis genital tract infections in males and females. These US Food and Drug Administration (FDA)-cleared and recommended tests can be collected via vaginal or cervical swabs from females and first-catch urine from females or males.[8] Compared with vaginal and cervical specimens, first-catch urine may detect up to 10% fewer infections among females.[9–11] Vaginal swabs are preferred for female screening, although urine is still recommended.[9,10,12–15] Urine is preferred for male urethral screening.[8] Rectal and oropharyngeal NAATs are not FDA cleared, but are recommended by the CDC based on increased sensitivity and ease of specimen transport and processing. This testing is available commercially and most reference laboratories have already performed internal validation for Clinical Laboratory Improvement Amendments (CLIA) approval; clinicians should discuss testing availability with their local laboratories.[8]

The use and acceptability for self-collected swab testing has been described in females as young as 12 years of age and is potentially cost saving in this group.[16–21] In a recent study of STI testing using clinic-based, self-collected vaginal swabs among 310 first-year female college students, 98% of students found it easy or very easy to understand collection instructions and 93% found it easy or very easy to collect the specimen. Among all females, self-collected specimens were preferred over clinician-collected specimens, and the majority of females noted that self-collection made them feel comfortable and in control and that they were taking care of their health.[22] Currently, multiple FDA-cleared NAAT platforms can be used for patient-collected vaginal swabs in a clinical setting.[8]

The CDC, the US Preventive Services Task Force (USPSTF), and the American Academy of Pediatrics (AAP) recommend routine annual chlamydia screening for sexually active females less than 25 years of age.[7,23,24] The CDC and AAP also recommend that clinicians should consider chlamydia screening in sexually active, heterosexual young males in clinical settings with higher chlamydia prevalence (including adolescent primary care clinics, correctional facilities, and STI clinics).

The recommendation for routine chlamydia screening remains unchanged for MSM based on most current guidelines, but more frequent screening at 3- to 6-month intervals is indicated for MSM, including those with human immunodeficiency virus (HIV) infection, based on risk factors in patients or their partners (see Special Populations: Men Who Have Sex With Men).

Treatment and Management

Recommended and alternative chlamydia treatments are outlined in **Table 1**. Recent studies suggest that doxycycline is marginally superior to azithromycin in treating genital chlamydia. Data from several studies and a metaanalysis show pooled cure rates of 97.5% for doxycycline versus 94.4% for azithromycin.[25–27] A recent randomized, controlled trial of males and females 12 to 21 years of age in a youth detention setting evaluated chlamydia directly observed therapy with doxycycline versus azithromycin. Treatment failure occurred in 5 of 155 individuals treated with azithromycin and none of the 155 individuals treated with doxycycline (cure rates of 97% and 100%, respectively.)[28] However, in settings in which directly observed therapy would not be feasible, that is, an office setting, single-dose azithromycin is still a highly effective and appropriate treatment option with a high cure rate.[29]

As mentioned, although routine oropharyngeal screening is not recommended, chlamydia can be transmitted sexually from oral to genital sites and should be treated if detected.[30,31] The efficacy of any of the alternative regimens is unknown for this indication.[7] Last, more recent retrospective studies including a systematic review and metaanalysis have raised some concern about the efficacy of single-dose azithromycin compared with doxycycline for rectal chlamydia infections.[32–34] More studies are needed comparing the 2 regimens before definitive recommendations can be made.[7]

Secondary to high reinfection rates, retesting in 3 months after chlamydia treatment is indicated in males and females.[35–37] NAAT testing should not be performed any sooner than approximately 1 month postinfection secondary to residual chlamydial DNA or RNA despite appropriate therapy.[7] Sexual partners in the past 60 days before diagnosis should be evaluated and treated. Or, if the last sexual exposure was more than 60 days before the onset of symptoms or diagnosis, the most recent sex partner should be treated. Partners should avoid sexual intercourse for at least 7 days after treatment to avoid reinfection.[7]

NEISSERIA GONORRHOEAE INFECTIONS

In the United States, gonorrhea is the second most frequently reported communicable disease after chlamydia.[1] N gonorrhoeae has evolved to resist each single antimicrobial agent used formerly as first-line therapy and cephalosporin resistance with accompanying treatment failures have been described worldwide (although not yet in the United States).[38–40] In a 2013 report, CDC designated N gonorrhoeae as antibiotic resistance threat level "urgent."[41]

Clinical Manifestations

N gonorrhoeae typically infects mucous membranes and may remain localized but can disseminate. Manifestations include urethritis, epididymitis, proctitis, conjunctivitis, cervicitis, PID, pharyngitis, and disseminated infection. Vertical transmission from infected mothers to their infants occurs. Gonorrhea can also increase rates of HIV sexual transmission up to 5-fold.[42]

Oral sex is highly prevalent among youth and prevalence of pharyngeal gonorrhea has increased in parallel. In 2 Los Angeles STI clinics, 65% of patients 15 to 24 years of age reported having oral sex and prevalence of pharyngeal gonorrhea in this group was 6%, compared with 7% for urogenital gonorrhea.[43]

Table 1
Recommended and alternative treatments for the major STDs in adolescents greater than 45 kg

Infection	Recommended Treatments	Alternative Treatments
Syphilis		
Primary, secondary or early latent (<1 y)	Benzathine penicillin G 50,000 units/kg IM once, up to adult dose of 2.4 million units	No specific alternative regimens exist.
Late latent (>1 y) or latent of unknown duration	Benzathine penicillin G 50,000 units/kg IM (up to adult dose of 2.4 million units) for 3 doses at 1 wk intervals (up to total adult dose of 7.2 million units)	No specific alternative regimens exist.
Gonorrhea		
Urogenital, pharyngeal and rectal	Ceftriaxone 250 mg IM once *plus* Azithromycin 1 g orally once	**Note: Use of an alternative regimen for pharyngeal gonorrhea should be followed by a test-of-cure 14 d after treatment.[a]** If ceftriaxone is *not* available: Cefixime 400 mg orally once[b] *plus* Azithromycin 1 g orally once *or in case of azithromycin allergy* Doxycycline[c] 100 mg orally 2 times a day for 7 d **For azithromycin allergy:** **Ceftriaxone 250 mg IM once *plus*** **Doxycycline[c] 100 mg orally 2 times a day for 7 d** **For cephalosporin allergy or IgE-mediated penicillin allergy:** **Gemifloxacin 320 mg orally once *or*** **Gentamicin 240 mg IM once** ***plus*** **Azithromycin 2 g orally once**
Conjunctival	Ceftriaxone 1 g IM once *plus* **Azithromycin 1 g orally once**, *plus* consider lavage of infected eye with saline solution once	No specific alternative regimens exist.
Chlamydia		
Urogenital, pharyngeal[d] and rectal[e]	Azithromycin 1 g orally once *or* Doxycycline[c] 100 mg orally 2 times a day for 7 d *or* Doxycycline hyclate[c] delayed-release tabs, 200 mg orally once daily for 7 d[f,g]	Erythromycin base 500 mg orally 4 times a day for 7 d[h] *or* Erythromycin ethylsuccinate 800 mg orally 4 times a day for 7 d[h] *or* Levofloxacin[i] 500 mg orally once a day for 7 d *or* Ofloxacin[i] 300 mg orally 2 times a day for 7 d

(continued on next page)

Table 1
(continued)

Infection	Recommended Treatments	Alternative Treatments
Trichomoniasis	Metronidazole 2 g orally once *or* Tinidazole 2 g orally once	Metronidazole[j] 500 mg orally 2 times a day for 7 d
Genital herpes simplex virus		
First clinical episode[k]	Acyclovir 400 mg orally 3 times a day for 7–10 d *or* Acyclovir 200 mg orally 5 times a day for 7–10 d *or* Valacyclovir 1 g orally 2 times a day for 7–10 d *or* Famciclovir[l] 250 mg orally 3 times a day for 7–10 d	
Recurrent disease (episodic therapy)	Acyclovir 400 mg orally 3 times a day for 5 d *or* Acyclovir 800 mg orally 2 times a day for 5 d *or* Acyclovir 800 mg orally 3 times a day for 2 d *or* Valacyclovir 500 mg orally 2 times a day for 3 d *or* Valacyclovir 1 g orally once a day for 5 d *or* Famciclovir[l] 125 mg orally 2 times a day for 5 d *or* Famciclovir[l] 1 g orally 2 times a day for 1 d *or* Famciclovir[l] 500 mg orally once, followed by 250 mg orally 2 times a day for 2 d	
Recurrent disease (suppressive therapy)	Acyclovir 400 mg orally 2 times a day *or* Valacyclovir 500 mg orally once a day *or* Valacyclovir 1 g orally once a day *or* Famciclovir[l] 250 mg orally 2 times a day	
Anogenital human papillomavirus		
External or perianal	Urethral meatus	Vaginal[p], cervical[q] or intraanal[r]

(continued on next page)

Table 1
(continued)

Infection	Recommended Treatments	Alternative Treatments
Provider administered • Cryotherapy with liquid nitrogen or cryoprobe. Repeat applications every 1–2 wk if necessary *or* • Surgical removal *or* • TCA or BCA 80% −90%. Apply small amount only to warts. Allow to dry. If excess amount applied, powder with talc, baking soda or liquid soap. Repeat weekly if necessary. Patient Applied • Imiquimod 5% cream[m]—apply once daily at bedtime 3 times a week for up to 16 wk; wash treatment area with soap and water 6–10 h after application *or* • **Imiquimod 3.75% cream[m]—apply once daily at bedtime every day for up to 16 wk; wash treatment area with soap and water 6–10 h after application** *or* • Podofilox 0.5% solution or gel[n]—apply 2 times a day for 3 d, followed by 4 d of no therapy, 4 cycles maximum; total wart area should not exceed 10 cm^2 and total volume applied daily not to exceed 0.5 mL *or* • Sinecatechins 15% ointment[o]—applied 3 times a day for up to 16 wk; do not wash off	• Cryotherapy with liquid nitrogen *or* • Surgical removal	• Cryotherapy with liquid nitrogen *or* • Surgical removal *or* • TCA or BCA 80%-90%: apply small amount only to warts; allow to dry; if excess amount applied, powder with talc, baking soda or liquid soap; repeat weekly if necessary

Revisions from the prior 2010 Centers for Disease Control and Prevention (CDC) STD Treatment Guidelines are emphasized in bold. See complete CDC Guidelines for management in pregnancy and in HIV infection.

Abbreviations: BCA, bichloroacetic acid; IgE, immunoglobulin E; IM, intramuscular; STD, sexually transmitted disease; TCA, trichloroacetic acid.

[a] Test of cure is no longer necessary in cases of uncomplicated urogenital or rectal gonorrhea treated with recommended or alternative regimens.

[b] Cefixime is not appropriate for pharyngeal gonococcal infections. See text.

[c] Doxycycline is not recommended during pregnancy or lactation.

[d] The efficacy of any of the *alternative* regimens is unknown for pharyngeal chlamydia; only recommended regimens should be used. See text.

[e] The efficacy of single-dose azithromycin compared with doxycycline for rectal chlamydia infections has yet to be studied in large trials. See text.

[f] This newer formulation comes in delayed-release 50 and 200 mg tabs and seems to be as effective as generic doxycycline with lower frequency of gastrointestinal side effects. Cost may be prohibitive for patients (approximately $340 for a 7-day course; in comparison, 7-day course of generic doxycycline ranges from $33–70).

[g] Thomson Reuters Micromedex Clinical Evidence Solutions [Internet]. Thomson Reuters; c2016. RED BOOK drug references; c2016 [cited 2016 Feb 11]. Available from: http://thomsonreuters.com/products_services/healthcare/healthcare_products/clinical_deci_support/micromedex_clinical_evidence_sols/med_safety_solutions/red_book/.

[h] If patient cannot tolerate high-dose erythromycin, change to lower dose for longer (refer to CDC Guidelines for details).

[i] Quinolones are not recommended for use in patients less than 18 years of age and are contraindicated in pregnancy.

[j] Regimen of 7 days of metronidazole may be more effective than single dose metronidazole in females coinfected with trichomoniasis and human immunodeficiency virus (HIV).

ᵏ Treatment can be extended if healing is incomplete after 10 days of therapy.
ˡ Famciclovir efficacy and safety has not established in patients less than 18 years of age.
ᵐ May weaken condoms and vaginal diaphragms. Data from studies of humans are limited regarding use of imiquimod in pregnancy, but animal data suggest imiquimod poses low risk.
ⁿ Podofilox is contraindicated in pregnancy.
ᵒ Sinecatechins are not recommended for HIV-infected persons, immunocompromised persons, or persons with clinical genital herpes. Safety of sinecatechins in pregnancy is unknown.
ᵖ Cryoprobe is not recommended secondary to risk for vaginal perforation and fistula formation.
ᑫ Exophytic cervical warts warrant biopsy to exclude high-grade squamous intraepithelial lesions before treatment is initiated. Management should include consultation with a specialist.
ʳ Many persons with anal warts may also have them in the rectal mucosa. Inspect rectal mucosa by digital examination or anoscopy. Management should include consultation with a specialist.
Adapted from Massachusetts Department of Public Health, Summary of the 2015 CDC STD Treatment Guidelines. Available at: http://www.mass.gov/eohhs/docs/dph/cdc/std/ma-std-tx-guidelines-2016.pdf. Accessed September 14, 2016.

Diagnosis and Screening

Similar to that for *C trachomatis* (see *Chlamydia trachomatis* infections), optimal detection of genital tract infections caused by *N gonorrhoeae* in males and females is achieved with NAATs collected via cervical or vaginal swabs (either clinician or patient collected in a clinical setting) from females and first-catch urine from females or males.[8] Clinicians should discuss testing availability with their local laboratories. Similar to chlamydia, the CDC, AAP, and USPSTF recommend routine gonorrhea screening for sexually active females less than 25 years of age.

The recommendation for routine gonorrhea screening remains unchanged for MSM based on most current guidelines, but more frequent screening at 3- to 6-month intervals is indicated for MSM, including those with HIV infection, based on risk factors in patients or their partners (see Special Populations: Men Who Have Sex With Men).

Treatment and Management

Recommended and alternative gonorrhea treatments are outlined in **Table 1**. Dual therapy is recommended to improve treatment efficacy and potentially slow the emergence and spread of cephalosporin resistance. Importantly, doxycycline is no longer recommended as part of dual therapy based on the substantially higher prevalence of gonococcal resistance to tetracycline.[7] Ideally, patients should receive dual therapy simultaneously and under direct observation in the clinic. If a prescription is given for azithromycin, it is critical to review with the patient the importance of dual therapy and that the azithromycin prescription should be filled and taken as soon as possible. If ceftriaxone is not available, then single-dose oral cefixime can be given in addition to azithromycin; however, this regimen is not appropriate for pharyngeal infections because cefixime has limited treatment efficacy for oral infections (92.3% cure [95% confidence interval, 74.9%–99.1%] compared with 97.5% cure [95% confidence interval, 95.4%–99.8%] in anogenital infections).[44,45]

A test of cure is only needed for individuals with pharyngeal gonorrhea treated with an alternative regimen; either culture or NAAT should be performed 14 days after treatment and any positive testing should be followed by antimicrobial susceptibility testing. Secondary to high reinfection rates, retesting in 3 months after therapy is indicated.[35,36] Sexual partners in the past 60 days before diagnosis should be evaluated and treated. Or, if the last sexual exposure was more than 60 days before onset of symptoms or diagnosis, the most recent sex partner should be treated. Partners should avoid sexual intercourse for at least 7 days after treatment to avoid reinfection.[7]

For those with cephalosporin or immunoglobulin E–mediated penicillin allergy, options are limited but include intramuscular gentamicin or oral gemifloxacin plus azithromycin based on a noncomparative randomized trial and in vitro studies.[46,47] Unfortunately, there is a current shortage of gemifloxacin in the United States; although the FDA approved a generic formulation in June 2015, it is unclear when this will become more available. Clinicians can find updates on the availability of gemifloxacin online via the CDC.[48]

Treatment Failures

Treatment failure should be considered in (1) persons whose symptoms do not resolve within 3 to 5 days after appropriate treatment and report no sexual contact during the posttreatment follow-up period and (2) persons with a positive test-of-cure (ie, positive culture ≥72 hours or positive NAAT ≥7 days after receiving recommended treatment) when no sexual contact is reported during the posttreatment follow-up period. In the adolescent population, a patient who is reinfected from an untreated or partially treated partner is the most commonly encountered situation rather than a case of resistant gonorrhea. If this situation is suspected, a careful history should be obtained and the patient should be retreated with ceftriaxone and azithromycin.[7] Clinicians should ensure that the patient's sex partners from the preceding 60 days are evaluated promptly with culture and presumptively treated using the same regimen used for the patient. A test of cure with a simultaneous NAAT at relevant clinical sites should be obtained 7 to 14 days after retreatment. It should be emphasized with the patient that he or she should abstain from sex for at least 1 week after treatment to avoid reinfection or transmission to a new partner.

In contrast, if treatment failure is truly suspected, clinicians should obtain relevant clinical specimens, including both NAAT and culture, and contact the local health department for guidance before retreatment.

TREPONEMA PALLIDUM INFECTIONS

Syphilis is caused by the spirochete *T pallidum* and is divided into stages (primary, secondary, latent, and tertiary) to guide management. As mentioned, there is a current epidemic of syphilis specifically in young MSM of color. Over time, there has been a 50% increase in HIV and a 200% increase in syphilis in this group.[1] In addition, a recent CDC *Morbidity and Mortality Weekly Report* alerted clinicians to an outbreak of ocular syphilis (a manifestation of neurosyphilis) in the Western United States in late 2014/early 2015, which has been of particular concern.[49,50]

Clinical Manifestations

Symptoms of syphilis depend on the stage and duration of infection; asymptomatic patients may only be diagnosed via screening. Patients with primary syphilis may present with painless ulcers or chancres on the genitalia, extremities, or oral mucosa depending on the location of exposure. Secondary syphilis symptoms can include skin rash, mucocutaneous lesions, and lymphadenopathy; tertiary syphilis presents with cardiac, neurologic, or gummatous manifestations decades after initial infection. Neurosyphilis can occur at any stage of disease.

As mentioned, 12 cases of ocular syphilis (including uveitis associated with rapidly progressive ocular symptoms and blindness) were initially identified in Seattle, Washington, and San Francisco, California, between December 2014 and March 2015. As of the latest update in March 2016, more than 200 cases have been reported from a total of 20 states. Most cases have been among HIV-positive MSM with a few cases in

HIV-negative patients including heterosexual males and females.[51] Although this outbreak has not yet affected adolescents, considering the syphilis epidemic in young MSM of color, clinicians should remain vigilant for this manifestation.

Diagnosis and Screening

Syphilis diagnosis requires both nontreponemal (eg, Venereal Disease Research Laboratory or rapid plasma reagin) and treponemal (eg, fluorescent treponemal antibody absorbed tests, the *T pallidum* passive particle agglutination assay, or enzyme immunoassay) testing. Because false-positive nontreponemal testing occurs in some situations (including pregnancy, autoimmune disease, HIV, and others), patients should always receive confirmatory treponemal testing.[7]

A growing number of clinical laboratories are screening samples initially using treponemal rather than nontreponemal tests, typically by enzyme immunoassay or chemiluminescence immunoassays, called the reverse screening algorithm. Such testing can be automated (in contrast, rapid plasma reagin is a manual test), has high sensitivity, and is optimal for populations with high prevalence of disease. In contrast, reverse screening cannot distinguish previous from new disease or treated from untreated disease, and secondary treponemal confirmation is required. False-positive initial treponemal results can occur in low-prevalence populations. Clinicians should be aware of the testing options at their institutions, and if reverse algorithm screening is available, they must be able to receive all treponemal and nontreponemal testing results to interpret the test results appropriately.[52] Of note, in 2014, the FDA granted a CLIA waiver for the Syphilis Health Check, a point-of-care test allowing for rapid screening in multiple clinical settings.[53] Local health departments and infectious diseases specialists can be contacted for discussion regarding testing availability and the most appropriate testing methodologies based on local epidemiology.

Patients with ocular symptoms consistent with syphilis should have serologic testing for syphilis in addition to immediate ophthalmologic evaluation and examination of the cerebrospinal fluid. Clinicians should contact their local health departments for guidance regarding suspected ocular syphilis cases.[50]

Treatment and Management

Syphilis treatments are outlined in **Table 1**. Of note, no adolescent or young adult-specific data exist. Primary and secondary syphilis-infected patients should be evaluated clinically and serologically for treatment failure at 6 and 12 months; those with latent syphilis should be evaluated clinically and serologically for treatment failure at 6, 12, and 24 months. Those with suspected neurosyphilis should be managed in collaboration with an infectious diseases specialist. In cases of suspected ocular syphilis, clinicians should contact their local health departments for discussion and guidance within 24 hours of diagnosis.[7]

TRICHOMONAS VAGINALIS INFECTIONS

Trichomoniasis is caused by the parasite *T vaginalis* and is the most prevalent nonviral STI in the United States. Although both males and females can be infected, this organism affects black females specifically (13% compared with 1.8% of non-Hispanic white females).[7] Infection may increase HIV acquisition risk by up to 3-fold, and it is particularly important in those coinfected with HIV based on studies of females 18 to 61 years of age: treatment can reduce genital HIV-1 shedding even in those not on antiretroviral therapy.[54–57] Therefore, sexually active HIV-positive females should be screened for trichomoniasis at care entry and then at least annually thereafter. The AAP recommends considering screening females at higher risk of infection.[58]

Clinical Manifestations

Most patients with trichomoniasis have few to no symptoms, and untreated infections can last for months or years. Symptoms in females include diffuse, malodorous or yellow-green vaginal discharge with or without vulvar irritation, and vaginitis or cervicitis on examination. Males may have urethritis, epididymitis, or prostatitis.

Diagnosis and Screening

All symptomatic individuals, particularly those with high-risk sexual behaviors, should be tested for trichomoniasis. Data are lacking on whether screening and treatment for asymptomatic trichomoniasis in high-prevalence settings or in persons at high risk can definitively reduce any adverse health events and health disparities or reduce community burden of infection.[58]

NAAT has the highest sensitivity and acceptable specificity for diagnosis of trichomoniasis and is available for females only from vaginal, endocervical, or urine specimens; however, the APTIMA assay may be used with male urine or urethral swabs if validated per CLIA regulations. The CLIA-waived point-of-care OSOM Trichomonas Rapid Test (Sekisui Diagnostics, Framingham, MA) relies on immunochromatographic antigen detection of *T vaginalis* in vaginal secretions, provides results in 10 minutes and has a sensitivity of 82% to 95% and specificity of 97% to 100%. The Affirm VP III (Becton Dickinson, Sparks, MD) is a DNA hybridization probe test that evaluates for *T vaginalis*, *Gardnerella vaginalis*, and *Candida albicans* in vaginal secretions. The trichomonas test sensitivity is 63% and specificity is 99.9%, and results are typically available in 45 minutes. The DNA hybridization probe test or culture have lower sensitivity and specificity and are not recommended as first-line screening tests if amplified molecular detection methods are available.[7] The microscopic evaluation of wet preparations (wet mount) is the most common method for *T vaginalis* diagnosis because of convenience and relatively low cost. However, it requires immediate specimen evaluation for optimal results, and has suboptimal sensitivity (51%–65% in vaginal specimens; even lower in male urethral, urine, or semen specimens).

Treatment and Management

Recommended and alternative trichomoniasis treatments are outlined in **Table 1**. Secondary to high reinfection rates, patient retesting in 3 months is indicated.[35,36]

HERPES SIMPLEX VIRUS INFECTIONS

Genital herpes is a chronic, life-long viral infection of 2 types: herpes simples virus (HSV)1 and HSV2. Most cases of recurrent genital herpes are caused by HSV2; however, HSV1 is becoming more prominent as a cause of first-episode genital herpes. Recent studies have supported the increase and/or stability in the rates of oral sex behaviors in both male and female adolescents and adults.[59–61] Over the last decade, HSV1 seroprevalence has decreased, leaving young people more susceptible to HSV disease and incident HSV1 infections at sexual debut. HSV1 now causes most first genital HSV episodes in young adults, specifically young females and MSM.[62]

Clinical Manifestations

Patients with HSV infection may have vesicular or ulcerative anogenital or oral lesions, but may also have episodes of asymptomatic viral shedding, which is much more frequent for genital HSV2 than for HSV1. Those with newly acquired disease can also have fever, malaise, and lymphadenopathy. Neonates can acquire devastating disease from vertical transmission. HSV2 also increases the risk of HIV acquisition.

Diagnosis and Screening

Cell culture or DNA polymerase chain reaction (PCR) are preferred for diagnosis in those with lesions. Although culture is highly specific, it is insensitive, may have a slow turnaround time, and testing is qualitative. PCR is highly sensitive and specific, type specific, automated, has a rapid turnaround time, and can be quantitative. It is the test of choice for central nervous system or systemic infections (including neonatal disease). Resistance testing can be done on culture but not on PCR. Importantly, failure to detect HSV by culture or PCR (especially in the absence of lesions) does not rule out HSV, because viral shedding is intermittent. Other tests, including the Tzanck preparation or direct immunofluorescence, have low sensitivity and/or specificity and are not recommended.

Serology with glycoprotein immunoglobulin G testing is type specific and accurate with sensitivities (HSV2) of 80% to 98%, although false-negatives may occur in early disease. The HerpeSelect HSV1 ELISA (Focus Diagnostics, Cypress, CA) is insensitive for detection of HSV1 antibody. The HerpeSelect HSV2 Elisa may have high false positives. HSV immunoglobulin M serology is not useful because is not type specific and may be positive during recurrent oral/genital episodes.

Because nearly all HSV2 infections are acquired sexually, the presence of HSV2 antibody implies anogenital infection. In contrast, the presence of HSV1 antibody alone is difficult to interpret because many individuals with positive testing may have been exposed in childhood with no implications for future disease or transmission to sexual partners. However, acquisition of genital HSV1 is increasing and can be asymptomatic. Lack of symptoms in a person who is HSV1 seropositive does not distinguish anogenital from orolabial or cutaneous infection, and regardless of site of infection, these persons remain at risk for acquiring HSV2.

Type-specific HSV serologic assays might be useful for (1) recurrent or atypical genital symptoms with negative HSV PCR or culture, (2) clinical diagnosis of genital herpes without laboratory confirmation, and (3) a patient whose partner has genital herpes. Screening for HSV1 and HSV2 in the general population is not indicated.

Treatment and Management

Recommended treatments for genital HSV infections are outlined in **Table 1**. Systemic antiviral therapy for HSV disease can treat symptomatic disease and control shedding, although famciclovir is less effective for the latter indication. Treatment also has no effect on latent virus, and it does not decrease risk of recurrence, frequency, or severity of episodes once it is discontinued. No topical therapy has been proven effective for HSV infection. In those with HIV, treatment decreases clinical symptoms but does not reduce HSV or HIV transmission risk to the uninfected partner; antivirals do not reduce risk of HIV acquisition in those who are HSV2 seropositive.

Daily suppressive therapy may be warranted for those with frequent episodes (>6 outbreaks per year) and can reduce the frequency of outbreaks by 70% to 80%. Treatment also is effective in patients with less frequent recurrences. Safety and efficacy has been studied in acyclovir (up to 6 years of documented experience) and valacyclovir and famciclovir up to 1 year. Any suppressive treatment should be reassessed yearly for necessity, as recurrences often decrease over time.[7]

Most persons with genital HSV remain undiagnosed and have mild or unrecognized infections, shedding virus intermittently. Most HSV transmission occurs via persons unaware of their infection. Thus, management must include counseling regarding the chronic nature of disease and the concept of asymptomatic shedding, rather than focusing solely on treating symptomatic episodes. The psychological effect of HSV infection can be substantial for patients. Strategies for HSV prevention in discordant couples include barrier methods (condoms), antivirals (for treatment and/or suppression), and avoidance of intercourse during symptomatic episodes. Disclosure can have a significant impact on disease acquisition. In a study of HSV1- and HSV2-infected patients aged 15 to 58 years (median, 26 years), those whose partners informed them that they had herpes had up to one-half of the risk of acquiring herpes compared with those with partners who did not inform them.[63]

HUMAN PAPILLOMAVIRUS INFECTIONS

Genital HPV is the most common STI in the United States and worldwide.[1,64] One-half of new infections occur in those 15 to 24 years of age, and 75% to 80% of sexually active adults will acquire genital tract HPV infection before the age of 50 years. Of note, 1 in 5 females with only 1 lifetime sexual partner has been infected with high-risk HPV.[1]

Clinical Manifestations

Although most infections are self-limited and/or asymptomatic, persistent infection can cause cervical cancer in females, as well as anogenital and oropharyngeal cancer, anogenital warts (AGW), and recurrent respiratory papillomatosis in males, females, and children. There are approximately 40 types of genital HPV, which can be categorized by their epidemiologic association with cervical cancer; the high-risk types are oncogenic while the low-risk types are primarily responsible for AGW.[65]

Diagnosis and Screening

Diagnosis of AGW is usually clinical. Acetic acid application is not a specific test for HPV infection. Therefore, the routine use of this procedure for screening to detect mucosal changes attributed to HPV infection is not recommended.[7] Routine cervical cancer screening should be performed in females 21 to 65 years and Pap testing every 3 years in those 21 to 29 years. HPV testing is never appropriate in any female younger than 21 years of age or in males, and should not be done as a screening test before vaccination, for STI screening, or for diagnosis of AGW.[66]

Treatment and Management

Recommended treatments for AGW are outlined in **Table 1**. There is no "best" or curative therapy and all have potential side effects and high recurrence rates, even with repeated therapy (20%–50% by 6 months).[7] The type of therapy is dictated by multiple factors including provider experience, patient preference and ability, size/number/location of warts, potential side effects, availability and expense. Although 10% to 30% of AGW may resolve on their own, persistent lesions can cause irritation and bleeding during intercourse, because lesions are typically friable. The removal of AGW likely reduces but is unlikely to completely eradicate infectivity.[7]

A diagnosis of AGW is not indicative of a partner's infidelity and it is unknown how long HPV remains contagious after treatment. Asymptomatic partners of patients with AGW do not need to be tested for HPV, and patients do not necessarily need to inform their future sex partners about a prior history of AGW, because this may not benefit the health of those partners.

Vaccination

The Advisory Committee on Immunization Practices now recommends immunization with HPV9. HPV9 is licensed for females 9 to 26 years of age. Although HPV9 is only licensed for males 9 to 15 years, the Advisory Committee on Immunization Practices has reviewed available bridging data and recommends HPV9 for all ages where HPV4 vaccine is recommended, including a routine vaccine for 13- to 21-year-old males and for 22- to 26-year-old MSM and HIV+ males and a permissive recommendation for other 22- to 26-year-old males. See Chapter 3 on the HPV Vaccine Update.

EMERGING ISSUES: *MYCOPLASMA GENITALIUM* INFECTIONS
Clinical Manifestations

M genitalium was first isolated in 1981 from urethral specimens of males with nongonococcal urethritis.[67] It is more common than gonorrhea but less common than chlamydia; similar to other STIs, prevalence varies based on the population studied.[7] In studies including young adults 18 to 24 years of age, *M genitalium* has been identified in approximately 15% to 20% of nongonococcal urethritis, 20% to 25% of nonchlamydial nongonococcal urethritis, and approximately 30% of persistent or recurrent urethritis cases.[68–71] It is unknown if *M genitalium* causes infertility or other anogenital tract disease besides urethritis in males; it can also be found in the rectum in asymptomatic males.

M genitalium's pathogenic role is less definitive in female reproductive tract disease because it can be found in the vagina, cervix, and endometrium of asymptomatic females. It has also been detected in 10% to 30% of clinical cervicitis cases.[72–78] Evidence suggests that *M genitalium* can cause PID, but less frequently than *C trachomatis*.[79,80]

Diagnosis and Screening

There is currently no FDA-approved diagnostic test for *M genitalium*, although many commercial laboratories have developed their own CLIA-certified PCR tests. Hologic, Inc (formerly Gen-Probe) recently launched its APTIMA *M genitalium* TMA assay and it is commercially available as an analyte-specific reagent platform.[81] Although FDA approval is pending, laboratories may obtain CLIA approval to use it as part of the APTIMA platform if they already use APTIMA NAATs (which are currently available for chlamydia, gonorrhea, and trichomoniasis testing). Clinicians are encouraged to contact their laboratories for information regarding availability of this assay.

Treatment and Management

In the absence of widely available testing, clinicians should consider treatment for *M genitalium* in cases of persistent or recurrent urethritis, cervicitis or PID unresponsive to standard empiric STI syndromic therapy. *M genitalium* lacks a cell wall; thus, antibiotics that target cell-wall biosynthesis, such as penicillins and cephalosporins, are ineffective. Cure rates with doxycycline range from 30% to 45% and for azithromycin, 40% to 87%.[25,26,82] The current recommended regimen is azithromycin 1 g orally once; however, there are emerging data regarding *M genitalium* azithromycin resistance. For suspected azithromycin treatment failures, clinicians may consider treatment with moxifloxacin 400 mg orally once daily for 7 to 14 days based on cure rates of 100% in initial reports.[83,84] Of note, data from Japan, Australia, and the United States show moxifloxacin treatment failures in some cases after the 7-day regimen.[85–88]

EMERGING ISSUES: HEPATITIS C INFECTIONS

Hepatitis C virus (HCV) is not efficiently transmitted sexually except in those with HIV. Incidence has been increasing in HIV+ MSM in the United States and Europe.[7] In the United States, a significant increase in new HCV infections, including in adolescents, has been noted concurrently with the drug use epidemic. In 2013, among all age groups, those aged 20 to 29 years had the highest rate (2.01 cases per 100,000 population) of acute disease.[1]

Clinical Manifestations

Those with acute HCV are usually asymptomatic or have mild symptoms. Chronic HCV develops in 70% to 85% of these patients and 60% to 70% of those with chronic disease develop active hepatitis. Chronic HCV may progress to cirrhosis and hepatocellular carcinoma.[7]

Diagnosis and Screening

The CDC and the USPSTF recommend HCV screening for those born between 1945 and 1965, with past or current injection or intranasal drug use, receiving a blood transfusion before 1992, on long-term hemodialysis, born to a mother with HCV infection, with an unregulated tattoo, or other related exposures. It is also now recommended to perform at least annual HCV screening for MSM because sexual transmission of HCV can occur, especially among MSM with HIV infection. An FDA-cleared HCV antibody test should be used first (ie, immunoassay, enzyme immunoassay) followed by NAAT if results are positive. Of note, antibody false negativity can occur in HIV-positive patients with a low CD4 counts and NAAT is particularly important in those cases.[7]

Treatment and Management

Any patient with positive HCV testing should be evaluated by specialists (typically infectious diseases physicians and/or gastroenterologists) for counseling and management. Therapy is available for HCV disease and can be curative. Vaccination against hepatitis A and B is also recommended. Specific recommendations for HCV management and treatment are available from the American Association for the Study of Liver Diseases and the Infectious Disease Society of America.[89]

SPECIAL POPULATIONS: MEN WHO HAVE SEX WITH MEN, WOMEN WHO HAVE SEX WITH WOMEN, AND TRANSGENDER INDIVIDUALS
Men Who Have Sex with Men

Recommendations for routine annual HIV screening, syphilis serologic testing, and chlamydia and gonorrhea screening remain unchanged for MSM based on most current guidelines. More frequent STI screening (ie, for syphilis, gonorrhea, and chlamydia) at 3- to 6-month intervals is indicated for MSM, including those with HIV infection, if risk behaviors persist in patients or their partners.

Studies in the 1980s and 1990s have shown increases in oral sex among heterosexual individuals, MSM, and adolescents.[90–93] In MSM, there was a decline in anal intercourse as a response to the HIV epidemic and studies show that recent sexual contacts reported by MSM are more likely to be orogenital or non–ano-penetrative.[94] Thus, it is critical to obtain a careful history about the type of sex (eg, oral, anal, or vaginal) and screen for STIs at all potentially exposed sites using NAAT testing to optimize sensitivity and specificity.

Women Who Have Sex With Women

Adolescent WSW may be at increased risk for STI and HIV acquisition based on reported risk factors.[95–99] Risk varies by the specific STI and sexual practice[100,101] and reported sexual identity does not always reflect sexual behavior. Studies show that 53% to 97% of self-identified WSW describe having male sexual contact in the past, and up to 28% have had male partners within the past year.[102–104] Thus, clinicians should ask about specific sex practices and partner types to identify the most appropriate screening types, modalities and sites for their patients.

WSW are at risk for acquiring HPV from partners of both sexes and should be offered routine cervical cancer screening and HPV vaccine as per current guidelines.[105] Transmission of HSV2 is inefficient in WSW, but they remain at risk for acquisition of both HSV2 and HSV1.[103,104] Transmission of bacterial infections between female partners, including syphilis, chlamydia, and bacterial vaginosis, is less clear. Bacterial vaginosis is generally common in women and especially in those with female partners,[106,107] but routine screening and partner therapy for such in WSW are not recommended at this time.

Transgender Individuals

Those who are transgender express a gender identity differing from the one corresponding with sex assignment at birth. In general, transgender women have a higher HIV prevalence compared with transgender men, but specific differences in other STIs have not yet been identified.[7] Clinicians should assess STI and HIV-related risks for their transgender patients based on current anatomy and specific sexual practices to determine the most appropriate screening.

SPECIAL ISSUES: EXPEDITED PARTNER THERAPY AND PREEXPOSURE PROPHYLAXIS
Expedited Partner Therapy

Expedited partner therapy (EPT) is the clinical practice of treating the sex partners of patients diagnosed with chlamydia or gonorrhea by providing prescriptions or medications to the patient to take to his/her partner without the health care provider first examining the partner. EPT is legal in most states but varies by type of STI authorized.[7] Information regarding state-specific EPT laws can be found on the CDC website (available: http://www.cdc.gov/std/ept/). The US EPT trials and a metaanalysis in females 14 years and older and males 16 years and older have shown reduced reinfection rates compared with patient referral strategies; across trials, reductions in chlamydia and gonorrhea prevalence at follow-up were 20% and 50%, respectively.[108–111] Several national organizations, including the AAP, endorse EPT use as a strategy to improve treatment and prevent reinfection in adolescents and young adults.[112–115]

Preexposure Prophylaxis for Human Immunodeficiency Virus Infection

HIV preexposure prophylaxis (PrEP) is the preventive use of daily oral antiretroviral therapy with a combination of tenofovir disoproxil fumarate and emtricitabine in HIV-negative patients at high risk for HIV acquisition. Although PrEP has been FDA approved in adults[116,117] and the CDC PrEP guidance targets this population,[118–120] the combination of tenofovir disoproxil fumarate and emtricitabine may be used off-label in those under 18 years of age. PrEP has been shown to be effective in reducing new HIV infections by 44% to 75% in adult MSM, heterosexuals, and injection drug users taking daily PrEP.[121–124] PrEP has also been found to be an acceptable and feasible intervention in young MSM.[125,126] Ongoing studies of PrEP in persons less than 18 years of age may lead to a PrEP indication in younger adolescents in the near future.[127] Barriers may exist to PrEP access, including parental consent requirement[128] and potential cost. PrEP may be paid for via Medicaid, participation in clinical trials, or industry-sponsored patient assistance programs.

SUMMARY

Adolescents are in a unique period of psychosocial and biologic development, placing them at high risk for STI acquisition and transmission. Some STIs are more prevalent among adolescents and young adults than among older men and women. Unfortunately, many providers who care for adolescents fail to discuss sexuality, even at health maintenance visits. Primary care visits present opportunities to educate adolescents on sexual health and development, to promote healthy relationships and to discuss prevention of STIs and HIV. (See Chapter 1 on Interviewing Adolescents about Sexual Matters). A confidential sexual history and STI screening are essential components of routine care for adolescents and young adults and updated guidelines should be used to guide prevention, screening, diagnosis, and management of STIs in this age group.

REFERENCES

1. Centers for Disease Control and Prevention (CDC). Sexually transmitted disease surveillance 2014. Atlanta (GA): US Department of Health and Human Services; 2015. Accessed January 18, 2016.
2. Spear LP. Adolescent neurodevelopment. J Adolesc Health 2013;52(2 Suppl 2): S7–13.
3. Panchaud C, Singh S, Reivelson D, et al. Sexually transmitted infections among adolescents in developed countries. Fam Plann Perspect 2000;32(1):24–32.
4. Mertz KJ, Finelli L, Levine WC, et al. Gonorrhea in male adolescents and young adults in Newark, New Jersey: implications of risk factors and patient preferences for prevention strategies. Sex Transm Dis 2000;27:201.
5. Boyer CB, Shafer MA, Teitle E, et al. Sexually transmitted disease in a health maintenance organization teen clinic: associations of race, partner's age, and marijuana use. Arch Pediatr Adolesc Med 1999;153:838.
6. Diclemente RJ, Wingood GM, Sionean C, et al. Association of adolescents' history of sexually transmitted disease (STD) and their current high risk behavior and STD status: a case for intensifying clinic-based prevention efforts. Sex Transm Dis 2002;29:503.
7. Centers for Disease Control and Prevention (CDC). Sexually transmitted diseases treatment guidelines, 2015. MMWR Recomm Rep 2015;64(3):1–138.
8. Papp JR, Schachter J, Gaydos CA, et al. Recommendations for the laboratory-based detection of Chlamydia trachomatis and Neisseria gonorrhoeae—2014. MMWR Recomm Rep 2014;63(2):1–17.
9. Schachter J, Chernesky MA, Willis DE, et al. Vaginal swabs are the specimens of choice when screening for Chlamydia trachomatis and Neisseria gonorrhoeae: results from a multicenter evaluation of the APTIMA assays for both infections. Sex Transm Dis 2005;32:725–8.
10. Michel CC, Sonnex C, Carne CA, et al. Chlamydia trachomatis load at matched anatomical sites: implications for screening strategies. J Clin Microbiol 2007;45: 1395–402.
11. Falk L, Coble BI, Mjörnberg PA, et al. Sampling for Chlamydia trachomatis infection—a comparison of vaginal, first-catch urine, combined vaginal and first-catch urine and endocervical sampling. Int J STD AIDS 2010;21:283–7.

12. Masek BJ, Arora N, Quinn N, et al. Performance of three nucleic acid amplification tests for detection of Chlamydia trachomatis and Neisseria gonorrhoeae by use of self-collected vaginal swabs obtained via n Internet-based screening program. J Clin Microbiol 2009;47:1663–7.

13. Shafer MA, Moncada J, Boyer CB, et al. Comparing first-void urine specimens, self-collected vaginal swabs, and endocervical specimens to detect *Chlamydia trachomatis* and *Neisseria gonorrhoeae* by a nucleic acid amplification test. J Clin Microbiol 2003;41:4395–9.

14. Schachter J, McCormack WM, Chernesky MA, et al. Vaginal swabs are appropriate specimens for diagnosis of genital tract infection with *Chlamydia trachomatis*. J Clin Microbiol 2003;41:3784–9.

15. Hsieh YH, Howell MR, Gaydos JC, et al. Preference among female army recruits for use of self-administered vaginal swabs or urine to screen for *Chlamydia trachomatis* genital infections. Sex Transm Dis 2003;30:769–73.

16. Serlin M, Shafer MA, Tebb K, et al. What sexually transmitted infection screening method does the adolescent prefer? Adolescents' attitudes towards first-void urine, self-collected vaginal swab, and pelvic examination. Arch Pediatr Adolesc Med 2002;156:588–91.

17. Hoebe CJ, Rademaker CW, Brouwers EE, et al. Acceptability of self-taken vaginal swabs and first-catch urine samples for the diagnosis of urogenital *Chlamydia trachomatis* and *Neisseria gonorrhoeae* with an amplified DNA assay in young women attending a public health sexually transmitted infection clinic. Sex Transm Dis 2006;33:491–5.

18. Graseck AS, Secura GM, Allsworth JE, et al. Home-screening compared with clinic-based screening for sexually transmitted infections. Obstet Gynecol 2010;115:745–52.

19. Cook RL, Østergaard L, Hillier SL, et al. Home screening for sexually transmitted infections in high risk young women: randomized controlled trial. Sex Transm Infect 2007;83:285–91.

20. Smith KJ, Cook RL, Ness RB. Cost comparisons between home- and clinic-based testing for sexually transmitted infections in high-risk young women. Infect Dis Obstet Gynecol 2007;2007:62467.

21. Huang W, Gaydos CA, Barnes MR, et al. Cost-effectiveness analysis of Chlamydia trachomatis screening via internet-based self-collected swabs compared to clinic-based sample collection. Sex Transm Dis 2011;38:815–20.

22. Fielder RL, Carey KB, Carey MP. Acceptability of STI testing using self-collected vaginal swabs among college women. J Am Coll Health 2013;61(1):46–53.

23. US Preventive Services Task Force. Screening for chlamydial infection: US preventive services task force recommendation statement. Ann Intern Med 2007; 147(2):128–34.

24. American Academy of Pediatrics (AAP). Committee on practice and ambulatory medicine, bright futures periodicity schedule workgroup. 2014 recommendations for pediatric preventive health care. Pediatrics 2014;133(3):568–70.

25. Schwebke JR, Rompalo A, Taylor S, et al. Re-evaluating the treatment of nongonococcal urethritis: emphasizing emerging pathogens—a randomized clinical trial. Clin Infect Dis 2011;52(2):163–70.

26. Manhart LE, Gillespie CW, Lowens MS, et al. Standard treatment regimens for nongonococcal urethritis have similar but declining cure rates: a randomized controlled trial. Clin Infect Dis 2013;56(7):934–42.

27. Kong FY, Tabrizi SN, Law M, et al. Azithromycin versus doxycycline for the treatment of genital chlamydia infection: a meta-analysis of randomized controlled trials. Clin Infect Dis 2014;59(2):193–205.

28. Geisler WM, Uniyal A, Lee JY, et al. Azithromycin versus doxycycline for urogenital chlamydia trachomatis Infection. N Engl J Med 2015;373(26):2512–21.

29. Quinn TC, Gaydos CA. Treatment for chlamydia infection—doxycycline versus azithromycin. N Engl J Med 2015;373(26):2573–5.

30. Bernstein KT, Stephens SC, Barry PM, et al. Chlamydia trachomatis and Neisseria gonorrhoeae transmission from the oropharynx to the urethra among men who have sex with men. Clin Infect Dis 2009;49:1793–7.

31. Marcus JL, Kohn RP, Barry PM, et al. Chlamydia trachomatis and Neisseria gonorrhoeae transmission from the female oropharynx to the male urethra. Sex Transm Dis 2011;38:372–3.

32. Hathorn E, Opie C, Goold P. What is the appropriate treatment for the management of rectal Chlamydia trachomatis in men and women? Sex Transm Infect 2012;88:352–4.

33. Steedman NM, McMillan A. Treatment of asymptomatic rectal Chlamydia trachomatis: is single-dose azithromycin effective? Int J STD AIDS 2009;20:16–8.

34. Kong FY, Tabrizi SN, Fairley CK, et al. The efficacy of azithromycin and doxycycline for the treatment of rectal chlamydia infection: a systematic review and meta-analysis. J Antimicrob Chemother 2015;70(5):1290–7.

35. Peterman TA, Tian LH, Metcalf CA, et al. High incidence of new sexually transmitted infections in the year following a sexually transmitted infection: a case for rescreening. Ann Intern Med 2006;145(8):564–72.

36. Turner AN, Feldblum PJ, Hoke TH. Baseline infection with a sexually transmitted disease is highly predictive of reinfection during follow-up in Malagasy sex workers. Sex Transm Dis 2010;37(9):559–62.

37. Aghaizu A, Reid F, Kerry S, et al. Frequency and risk factors for incident and re-detected Chlamydia trachomatis infection in sexually active, young, multi-ethnic women: a community-based cohort study. Sex Transm Infect 2014;90(7):524–8.

38. Ohnishi M, Golparian D, Shimuta K, et al. Is Neisseria gonorrhoeae initiating a future era of untreatable gonorrhea? Detailed characterization of the first strain with high-level resistance to ceftriaxone. Antimicrob Agents Chemother 2011; 55:3538–45.

39. Unemo M, Golparian D, Nicholas R, et al. High-level cefixime- and ceftriaxone-resistant N. gonorrhoeae in France: novel penA mosaic allele in a successful international clone causes treatment failure. Antimicrob Agents Chemother 2012; 56:1273–80.

40. Cámara J, Serra J, Ayats J, et al. Molecular characterization of two high-level ceftriaxone-resistant Neisseria gonorrhoeae isolates detected in Catalonia, Spain. J Antimicrob Chemother 2012;67:1858–60.

41. Centers for Disease Control and Prevention (CDC). Antibiotic resistance threats in the United States, 2013. Available at www.cdc.gov/drugresistance/threat-report-2013/. Accessed December 21, 2015.

42. Cohen MS. Sexually transmitted diseases enhance HIV transmission: no longer a hypothesis. Lancet 1998;351(Suppl III):5–7.

43. Los Angeles County Department of Public Health. Sexually transmitted disease program. STD clinic morbidity report, Los Angeles county 2007. p. I-1–XVII-2.

44. Moran JS, Levine WC. Drugs of choice for the treatment of uncomplicated gonococcal infections. Clin Infect Dis 1995;20(Suppl 1):S47–65.

45. Newman LM, Moran JS, Workowski KA. Update on the management of gonor-rhea in adults in the United States. Clin Infect Dis 2007;44(Suppl 3):S84–101.
46. Kirkcaldy RD, Weinstock HS, Moore PC, et al. The efficacy and safety of genta-micin plus azithromycin and gemifloxacin plus azithromycin as treatment of un-complicated gonorrhea. Clin Infect Dis 2014;59(8):1083–91.
47. Tanaka M, Tunoe H, Mochida O, et al. Antimicrobial activity of gemifloxacin (SB-265805), a newer fluoroquinolone, against clinical isolates of Neisseria gonor-rhoeae, including fluoroquinolone-resistant isolates. Diagn Microbiol Infect Dis 2000;38(2):109–13.
48. Centers for Disease Control and Prevention (CDC): Gemifloxacin shortage. Avail-able at: www.cdc.gov/std/treatment/drugnotices/gemifloxacin.htm. Accessed April 25, 2016.
49. Woolston S, Cohen SE, Fanfair RN, et al. A Cluster of Ocular Syphilis Cases – Seattle, Washington, and San Francisco, California, 2014-2015. MMWR Re-comm Rep 2015;64(40):1150–1.
50. Clinical advisory: ocular syphilis in the United States. Division of STD Prevention, National Center for HIV/AIDS, Viral Hepatitis, STD and TB Prevention, Centers for Disease Control and Prevention, November 2015. Available at: http://www.cdc.gov/std/syphilis/clinicaladvisoryos2015.htm. Accessed November 15, 2016.
51. Centers for Disease Control and Prevention (CDC). Clinical advisory: ocular syphilis in the United States. Available at: http://www.cdc.gov/std/syphilis/clinical advisoryos2015.htm. Accessed April 15, 2016.
52. Centers for Disease Control and Prevention (CDC). Discordant results from reverse sequence syphilis screening—five laboratories, United States, 2006-2010. MMWR Morb Mortal Wkly Rep 2011;60(5):133–7.
53. US Food and Drug Administration (FDA). FDA News Release: DFA grants CLIA waiver expanding the availability of rapid screening test for syphilis, December 2014. Available at: http://www.fda.gov/NewsEvents/Newsroom/Press Announcements/ucm426843.htm. Accessed September 2, 2016.
54. Klinger EV, Kapiga SH, Sam NE, et al. A community-based study of risk factors for Trichomonas vaginalis infection among women and their male partners in Moshi urban district, northern Tanzania. Sex Transm Dis 2006;33:712–8.
55. McClelland RS, Sangare L, Hassan WM, et al. Infection with Trichomonas vag-inalis increases the risk of HIV-1 acquisition. J Infect Dis 2007;195:698–702.
56. Kissinger P, Amedee A, Clark RA, et al. Trichomonas vaginalis treatment re-duces vaginal HIV-1 shedding. Sex Transm Dis 2009;36:11–6.
57. Anderson BL, Firnhaber C, Liu T, et al. Effect of trichomoniasis therapy on genital HIV viral burden among African women. Sex Transm Dis 2012;39:638–42.
58. AAP Committee on Adolescence and Society for Adolescent Health and Medi-cine. Screening for nonviral sexually transmitted infections in adolescents and young adults. Pediatrics 2014;134:e302–11.
59. Aral SO, Patel DA, Holmes KK, et al. Temporal trends in sexual behaviors and sexually transmitted disease history among 18- to 39-year-old Seattle, Washing-ton residents: results of random digit-dial surveys. Sex Transm Dis 2005;32(11):710–7.
60. Mosher WD, Chandra A, Jones J. Sexual behavior and selected health mea-sures: men & women 15-44 years of age, United States, 2002. Adv Data 2005;362:1–55.
61. Copen CE, Chandra A, Martinez G. Prevalence and timing of oral sex with opposite-sex partners among females and males aged 15-24 years: United States, 2007-2010. Natl Health Stat Report 2012;56:1–14.

62. Kimberlin DW. The scarlet H. J Infect Dis 2014;209(3):315–7.
63. Wald A, Krantz E, Selke S, et al. Knowledge of partners' genital herpes protects against herpes simplex virus type 2 acquisition. J Infect Dis 2006;194(1):42–52.
64. Forman D, de Martel C, Lacey CJ, et al. Global burden of human papillomavirus and related diseases. Vaccine 2012;30(Suppl 5):F12–23.
65. Munoz N, Bosch FX, de Sanjose S, et al. Epidemiologic classification of human papillomavirus types associated with cervical cancer. N Engl J Med 2003;348: 518–27.
66. American Society for Colposcopy and Cervical Pathology. 2012 Updated Consensus Guidelines for Management of Abnormal Cervical Cancer Screening Tests and Cancer Precursors. Available at: http://www.asccp.org/guidelines. Accessed April 18, 2016.
67. Tully JG, Taylor-Robinson D, Cole RM, et al. A newly discovered mycoplasma in the human urogenital tract. Lancet 1981;1(8233):1288–91.
68. Totten PA, Schwartz MA, Sjostrom KE, et al. Association of Mycoplasma genitalium with nongonococcal urethritis in heterosexual men. J Infect Dis 2001; 183(2):269–76.
69. Mena L, Wang X, Mroczkowski TF, et al. Mycoplasma genitalium infections in asymptomatic men and men with urethritis attending a sexually transmitted diseases clinic in New Orleans. Clin Infect Dis 2002;35:1167–73.
70. Manhart LE, Holmes KK, Hughes JP, et al. Mycoplasma genitalium among young adults in the United States: an emerging sexually transmitted infection. Am J Public Health 2007;97(6):1118–25.
71. Taylor-Robinson D, Jensen JS. Mycoplasma genitalium: from chrysalis to multicolored butterfly. Clin Microbiol Rev 2011;24:498–514.
72. Falk L. The overall agreement of proposed definitions of mucopurulent cervicitis in women at high risk of chlamydia infection. Acta Derm Venereol 2010;09: 506–11.
73. Anagrius C, Lore B, Jensen JS. Mycoplasma genitalium: prevalence, clinical significance, and transmission. Sex Transm Infect 2005;81:458–62.
74. Falk L, Fredlund H, Jensen JS. Signs and symptoms of urethritis and cervicitis among women with or without Mycoplasma genitalium or Chlamydia trachomatis infection. Sex Transm Infect 2005;81:73–8.
75. Manhart LE, Critchlow CW, Holmes KK, et al. Mucopurulent cervicitis and Mycoplasma genitalium. J Infect Dis 2003;187(4):650–7.
76. Gaydos C, Maldeis NE, Hardick A, et al. Mycoplasma genitalium as a contributor to the multiple etiologies of cervicitis in women attending sexually transmitted disease clinics. Sex Transm Dis 2009;36(10):598–606.
77. Mobley VL, Hobbs MM, Lau K, et al. Mycoplasma genitalium infection in women attending a sexually transmitted infection clinic: diagnostic specimen type, co-infections, and predictors. Sex Transm Dis 2012;39(9):706–9.
78. Lusk MJ, Konecny P, Naing ZW, et al. Mycoplasma genitalium is associated with cervicitis and HIV infection in an urban Australian STI clinic population. Sex Transm Infect 2011;87(2):107–9.
79. Bjartling C, Osser S, Persson K. Mycoplasma genitalium and Chlamydia trachomatis in laparoscopically diagnosed pelvic inflammatory disease. STI & AIDS World Congress 2013 (Joint Meeting of the 20th ISSTDR and 14th IUSTI Meeting). Vienna, Austria, July 14–17, 2013.
80. Oakeshott P, Kerry S, Aghaizu A, et al. Randomised controlled trial of screening for Chlamydia trachomatis to prevent pelvic inflammatory disease: the POPI (prevention of pelvic infection) trial. BMJ 2010;340:c1642.

81. Centers for Disease Control and Prevention (CDC): *Mycoplasma genitalium* Questions & Answers. Available at: http://www.cdc.gov/std/tg2015/qa/myco plasma-genitaliumqa.htm. Accessed April 25, 2016.
82. Mena LA, Mroczkowski TF, Nsuami M, et al. A randomized comparison of azithromycin and doxycycline for the treatment of Mycoplasma genitalium-positive urethritis in men. Clin Infect Dis 2009;48(12):1649–54.
83. Jernberg E, Moghaddam A, Moi H. Azithromycin and moxifloxacin for microbiological cure of Mycoplasma genitalium infection: an open study. Int J STD AIDS 2008;19:676–9.
84. Bradshaw CS, Chen MY, Fairley CK. Persistence of *Mycoplasma genitalium* following azithromycin therapy. PLoS One 2008;3:e3618.
85. Terada M, Izumi K, Ohki E, et al. Antimicrobial efficacies of several antibiotics against uterine cervicitis caused by *Mycoplasma genitalium*. J Infect Chemother 2012;18(3):313–7.
86. Manhart LE, Khosropour CM, Gillespie CW, et al. Treatment outcomes for persistent Mycoplasma genitalium associated NGU: evidence of moxifloxacin treatment failures. STI & AIDS World Congress Joint Meeting of the 20th International Society for Sexually Transmitted Disease Research. Vienna, Austria, July 14–17, 2013.
87. Couldwell DL, Tagg KA, Jeoffreys NJ, et al. Failure of moxifloxacin treatment in *Mycoplasma genitalium* infections due to macrolide and fluoroquinolone resistance. Int J STD AIDS 2013;24(10):822–8.
88. Tagg KA, Jeoffreys NJ, Couldwell DL, et al. Fluoroquinolone and macrolide resistance-associated mutations in *Mycoplasma genitalium*. J Clin Microbiol 2013;51(7):2245–9.
89. American Association for the Study of Liver Diseases and the Infectious Disease Society of America. Recommendations for testing, managing and treating Hepatitis C. Available at: http://www.hcvguidelines.org. Accessed March 11, 2016.
90. Johnson AM, Wadsworth J, Wellings K, et al. The national survey of sexual attitudes and lifestyles. Oxford (United Kingdom): Blackwell Scientific Press; 1994.
91. Kinsey A, Pomeroy W, Martin C. Sexual behavior in the human male. Philadelphia: WB Saunders; 1948.
92. Kinsey A, Pomeroy W, Martin C, et al. Sexual behavior in the human female. Philadelphia: WB Saunders; 1953.
93. Gagnon JH, Simon W. Sexual scripting of oral genital contacts. Arch Sex Behav 1987;16(1):1–25.
94. Winkelstein W Jr, Samuel M, Padian NS, et al. The San Francisco Men's Health Study: III. Reduction in HIV transmission among homosexual/bisexual men, 1982-86. Am J Public Health 1987;77(6):685–9.
95. Muzny CA, Sunesara IR, Martin DH, et al. Sexually transmitted infections and risk behaviors among African American women who have sex with women: does sex with men make a difference? Sex Transm Dis 2011;38:1118–25.
96. Eisenberg M. Differences in sexual risk behaviors between college students with same-sex and opposite-sex experience: results from a national survey. Arch Sex Behav 2001;30:575–89.
97. Koh AS, Gomez CA, Shade S, et al. Sexual risk factors among selfidentified lesbians, bisexual women, and heterosexual women accessing primary care settings. Sex Transm Dis 2005;32:563–9.
98. Lindley L, Burcin M. STD diagnoses among sexually active female college students: does sexual orientation or gender of sex partner(s) make a difference? National STD Prevention Conference. Chicago, IL, March 10-13, 2008.

99. Goodenow C, Szalacha LA, Robin LE, et al. Dimensions of sexual orientation and HIV-related risk among adolescent females: evidence from a statewide survey. Am J Public Health 2008;98:1051–8.
100. Fethers K, Marks C, Mindel A, et al. Sexually transmitted infections and risk behaviours in women who have sex with women. Sex Transm Infect 2000;76: 345–9.
101. Marrazzo JM, Koutsky LA, Eschenbach DA, et al. Characterization of vaginal flora and bacterial vaginosis in women who have sex with women. J Infect Dis 2002;185:1307–13.
102. Diamant AL, Schuster MA, McGuigan K, et al. Lesbians' sexual history with men: implications for taking a sexual history. Arch Intern Med 1999;159:2730–6.
103. Xu F, Sternberg MR, Markowitz LE. Women who have sex with women in the United States: prevalence, sexual behavior and prevalence of herpes simplex virus type 2 infection-results from national health and nutrition examination survey 2001-2006. Sex Transm Dis 2010;37:407–13.
104. Marrazzo JM, Stine K, Wald A. Prevalence and risk factors for infection with herpes simplex virus type-1 and-2 among lesbians. Sex Transm Dis 2003;30:890–5.
105. Markowitz LE, Dunne EF, Saraiya M, et al. Human papillomavirus vaccination: recommendations of the Advisory Committee on Immunization Practices (ACIP). MMWR Recomm Rep 2014;63(RR-05):1–30.
106. Koumans EH, Sternberg M, Bruce C, et al. The prevalence of bacterial vaginosis in the United States, 2001-2004: associations with symptoms, sexual behaviors, and reproductive health. Sex Transm Dis 2007;34:864–9.
107. Evans AL, Scally AJ, Wellard SJ, et al. Prevalence of bacterial vaginosis in lesbians and heterosexual women in a community setting. Sex Transm Infect 2007; 83:470–5.
108. Trelle S, Shang A, Nartey L, et al. Improved effectiveness of partner notification for patients with sexually transmitted infections: systematic review. BMJ 2007; 334:354.
109. Golden MR, Whittington WL, Handsfield HH, et al. Effect of expedited treatment of sex partners on recurrent or persistent gonorrhea or chlamydial infection. N Engl J Med 2005;352:676–85.
110. Schillinger JA, Kissinger P, Calvet H, et al. Patient-delivered partner treatment with azithromycin to prevent repeated Chlamydia trachomatis infection among women – a randomized, controlled trial. Sex Transm Dis 2003;30:49–56.
111. Kissinger P, Mohammed H, Richardson-Alston G, et al. Patient-delivered partner treatment for male urethritis: a randomized, controlled trial. Clin Infect Dis 2005; 41:623–9.
112. American Medical Association. CSAPH Report 7-A-06 Expedited partner therapy (patient-delivered partner therapy): an update. Available at: www.ama-assn.org/resources/doc/csaph/a06csaph7-fulltext.pdf. Accessed February 10, 2016.
113. Committee Opinion No. 506: Expedited partner therapy in the management of gonorrhea and chlamydia by obstetrician-gynecologists. Obstet Gynecol 2011;118:761–6.
114. Hodge JG Jr, Pulver A, Hogben M, et al. Expedited partner therapy for sexually transmitted infections: assessing the legal environment. Am J Public Health 2008;98:238–43.
115. Burstein GR, Eliscu A, Ford K, et al. Expedited partner therapy for adolescents diagnosed with chlamydia or gonorrhea: a position paper of the society for adolescent medicine. J Adolesc Health 2009;45:303–9.

116. FDA. FDA approves first drug for reducing the risk of sexually acquired HIV infection. 2012. Available at: http://www.fda.gov/NewsEvents/Newsroom/Press Announcements/ucm312210.htm. Accessed February 10, 2016.
117. Holmes D. FDA paves the way for pre-exposure HIV prophylaxis. Lancet 2012; 380:325.
118. Centers for Disease Control and Prevention (CDC). Interim guidance: preexposure prophylaxis for the prevention of HIV infection in men who have sex with men. MMWR Morb Mortal Wkly Rep 2011;60:65–8.
119. Centers for Disease Control and Prevention (CDC). Interim guidance for clinicians considering the use of preexposure prophylaxis for the prevention of HIV infection in heterosexually active adults. MMWR Morb Mortal Wkly Rep 2012;61:586–9.
120. Centers for Disease Control and Prevention (CDC). Update to interim guidance for preexposure prophylaxis (PrEP) for the prevention of HIV infection: PrEP for injecting drug users. MMWR Morb Mortal Wkly Rep 2013;62:463–5.
121. Grant RM, Lama JR, Anderson PL, et al. Preexposure chemoprophylaxis for HIV prevention in men who have sex with men. N Engl J Med 2010;363(27):2587–99.
122. Baeten JM, Donnell D, Ndase P, et al. Antiretroviral prophylaxis for HIV prevention in heterosexual men and women. N Engl J Med 2012;367(5):399–410.
123. Thigpen MC, Kebaabetswe PM, Paxton LA, et al. Antiretroviral preexposure prophylaxis for heterosexual HIV transmission in Botswana. N Engl J Med 2012; 367(5):423–34.
124. Choopanya K, Martin M, Suntharasamai P, et al. Antiretroviral prophylaxis for HIV infection in injecting drug users in Bangkok, Thailand (the Bangkok Tenofovir Study): a randomized, double-blind, placebo-controlled phase 3 trial. Lancet 2013;381(9883):2083–90.
125. Hosek SG, Siberry G, Bell M, et al. The acceptability and feasibility of an HIV preexposure prophylaxis (PrEP) trial with young men who have sex with men. J Acquir Immune Defic Syndr 2013;62(4):447–56.
126. Mugwanya KK, Donnell D, Celum C, et al. Sexual behaviour of heterosexual men and women receiving antiretroviral pre-exposure prophylaxis for HIV prevention: a longitudinal analysis. Lancet Infect Dis 2013;13(12):1021–8.
127. Pace JE, Siberry GK, Hazra R, et al. Pre-exposure prophylaxis for adolescents and young adults at risk for HIV infection: is an ounce of prevention worth a pound of cure? Clin Infect Dis 2013;56:1149–55.
128. Culp L, Caucci L. State adolescent consent laws and implications for HIV Preexposure prophylaxis. Am J Prev Med 2013;44(1S2):S119–24.

Sex Trafficking of Minors

Jessica L. Moore, BA[a], Dana M. Kaplan, MD[b],
Christine E. Barron, MD[a,c],*

KEYWORDS

- Domestic minor sex trafficking (DMST)
- Commercial sexual exploitation of children (CSEC) • Sexual abuse
- Sexual exploitation • Sexually transmitted infection (STI)

KEY POINTS

- Youth involved in domestic minor sex trafficking (DMST) have serious immediate and long-term physical and mental health consequences.
- A coordinated multidisciplinary team response is needed.
- Standardized national medical protocols for DMST youth are needed to improve the prevention, identification, and effective interventions (medical and service provisions).

DEFINITIONS

Sex Trafficking

Sex trafficking is an increasingly recognized global health crisis affecting every country and region in the world. By definition, sex trafficking is the recruitment, harboring, transportation, provision, or obtaining of a person for the purpose of a commercial sex act in exchange for anything of value, by means of threat, force, fraud, or coercion.[1] Survivors include adults, adolescents, and children. The International Labor Organization estimates that 2.5 million adults and children are at risk for trafficking worldwide.[2]

Commercial Sexual Exploitation of Children

Commercial sexual exploitation of children (CSEC) is sex trafficking of children and is defined as the engagement of minors (<18 years of age) in sexual acts for items of value (eg, food, shelter, drugs, money). The identification of minors as victims does

Disclosure Statement: The authors have no commercial or financial conflicts of interest or funding sources.
[a] Department of Pediatrics, Aubin Child Protection Center, Hasbro Children's Hospital, 593 Eddy Street, Potter Building 005, Providence, RI 02903, USA; [b] Division of Child Abuse and Neglect, Department of Pediatrics, Staten Island University Hospital, 475 Seaview Avenue, Staten Island, NY 10305, USA; [c] Department of Pediatrics, The Warren Alpert Medical School of Brown University, 222 Richmond Street, Providence, RI 02903, USA
* Corresponding author. Aubin Child Protection Center, Hasbro Children's Hospital, 593 Eddy Street, Potter Building 005, Providence, RI 02903.
E-mail address: cbarron1@lifespan.org

Pediatr Clin N Am 64 (2017) 413–421
http://dx.doi.org/10.1016/j.pcl.2016.11.013
0031-3955/17/© 2016 Elsevier Inc. All rights reserved.
pediatric.theclinics.com

not require evidence of threat, force, fraud, or coercion.[1,3] Within this definition, sexual acts are broadly defined to include street-based and Internet-based sex, escorting, stripping, pornography, or any act completed for sexual purposes in any venue.[3]

CSEC occurs both internationally (international sex trafficking) and domestically (domestic minor sex trafficking [DMST]). These adolescents can be trafficked across national borders (transnational trafficking), or within a country, a state, or even within a single neighborhood.[3] Until recently, human trafficking and CSEC have been perceived to be problems that occur in other countries, or involving the trafficking of international minors when it occurs within the United States.[4] However, over the last several years there has been increasing recognition of a previously unidentified population of children who are US citizens or residents living in and sex trafficked within the United States; this is known as DMST.

Domestic Minor Sex Trafficking

As a subset of CSEC, DMST specifically involves US citizens or legal residents victimized within US borders.[3] It is conservatively estimated that approximately 150,000 to 300,000 US children are at risk for commercial sexual exploitation each year.[5,6] These minors have not been brought from other countries for the purpose of commercial sex acts, and are therefore not survivors of international sex trafficking.[7] This distinction is important as survivors of domestic sex trafficking differ significantly from survivors of international sex trafficking, including a higher association with poorer health outcomes (physical injuries, sexually transmitted infections [STIs]), histories of child physical and/or sexual abuse, alcohol/drug addiction, and reported suicidal ideations for domestic survivors.[8] This article focuses on issues related to DMST within the United States.

Minors involved in the commercial sex trade may erroneously be referred to as child prostitutes. The use of this terminology frames youth as criminals instead of correctly identifying them as vulnerable youth in need of support and services.[7] With greater awareness of this issue, there will continue to be an appropriate shift away from the disparaging paradigm of juvenile delinquent behavior to a conception of involved youth as survivors of child sexual abuse.

RISK
Epidemiology

Obtaining accurate figures for the prevalence and incidence of sex trafficking has been challenging given the hidden nature of these crimes, survivors denying involvement, lack of collaboration across multiple disciplines, and the application of different definitions and laws.[3] The incidence of DMST is thought to be underreported, similar to cases of child sex abuse, and in particular there is a paucity of reporting by male survivors.[3,7] Accurate identification may improve with a uniform approach to this problem across the country, including more frequent screening, especially in high-risk populations.

In general, all adolescents are at risk of attempted recruitment because the average age of entry into the commercial sex industry is reported to be 12 to 16 years.[5,9]

Normative Adolescent Psychosocial Development

Normal adolescent development involves the progression of independence from parents; peer relationships; sexual experimentation; intellectual advancement from concrete to abstract thinking; in combination with impulsivity, risk-taking behaviors, and a sense of invulnerability.[10] Traffickers prey on these normal adolescent vulnerabilities, thereby placing all adolescents at risk for DMST recruitment and subsequent involvement.

Risk Factors

Although all adolescents are at risk, some children are at heightened risk because of individual, family, and community factors.[11] According to the Institute of Medicine, children with a history of maltreatment, particularly sexual abuse,[12] are at especially high risk of exploitation, as are youth who come from dysfunctional families (eg, parental substance abuse, domestic violence). Histories of child protective services involvement, alcohol and substance use, and/or mental health disorders may play a role in a minor's involvement.[6,11,12] Runaway, homeless, and group home youth are also at high risk because they often come from environments with caregiver abandonment or impaired supervision, poverty, neglect, and abuse.[11,12] Children with these aforementioned risk factors are targeted by exploiters because of their emotional, physical, and financial vulnerabilities, and subsequent susceptibility to engage in risk-taking behaviors.

RECRUITMENT
Grooming

In child sexual abuse, the process by which a child molester overcomes a child's resistance to sex and elicits cooperation in a progressive manner is referred to as grooming.[13] In building this relationship, the molester may offer love and/or items to gain the trust of the child. Moreover, the act of grooming develops a relationship bonding perpetrators and youth.[13] The act of grooming is often used in the recruitment process for DMST. Traffickers may use manipulative strategies to seduce minors with promises of money, better lives, and/or love and security.[14,15] Commonly, the trafficker establishes a relationship with the adolescent similar to a romantic partner or friend.[16] Subsequent techniques, such as fear and coercion, are used to keep the involved youth from leaving. Notably, minors are not often physically restrained but are psychologically manipulated by their exploiters to continue their involvement. Same-age peers may act as recruiters, attempting to normalize these acts to other adolescents as a potential positive financial strategy.[16]

Survivor-Exploiter Dynamics

The relationship that develops between the minor and exploiter in DMST is similar to that seen in cases of intimate partner violence (IPV). The Power and Control Wheel developed by Pence and Paymar[17] for IPV is often used with minimal changes to show the similarities in the dynamics of establishing and maintaining relationships of survivors with perpetrators in DMST. These tactics eventually undermine the adolescent's ability to act autonomously, keeping involved youth under the control of their exploiters.[17]

In addition, a recruitment tactic of exploiters may be the provision of alcohol and/or illicit substances to minors. Over time, dependencies on substances are used by exploiters to maintain power and ensure the minor's continued involvement.[5,16]

Social Media

Social media plays an integral role in the complex dynamics of adolescent, recruitment and the solicitation of sex buyers/clients. Recruitment through social media is underscored by the role of peer recruiters.[18] Individuals whom involved youth consider friends may work as surrogate recruiters for traffickers by modeling this behavior and normalizing participation in sex trafficking. Social media is often the means through which recruiters prey on vulnerable youth by establishing a friendship or romantic relationship.[9,16]

The initial interaction between recruiter and involved youth may occur face to face, but social media sites are often used in the grooming process and, ultimately, to keep reinforcing the prospect of trafficking; this makes exiting from DMST an even greater challenge because several survivors may remain connected online.

Furthermore, the use of Internet sites, and specifically social media, is a well-documented method for the solicitation of clients.[9,16] Classified advertisement Web sites, such as Backpage.com, have been used to advertise sex services with minors.[9] Involved youth and/or exploiters are contacted by sex buyers and encounters are subsequently arranged.

IDENTIFICATION
Barriers to Care

There are numerous challenges associated with the identification of victimized or high-risk youth.[3,7] Many adolescents involved in DMST do not self-identify or present with confirmatory evidence (eg, found by law enforcement, known to have Internet pictures posted) of involvement. Thus, it is incumbent on medical providers to recognize possible indicators of involvement for victimized and vulnerable adolescents.

Many DMST survivors have an overwhelming distrust of authority figures based on their histories of child maltreatment, abandonment by caregivers, and prior interactions with child protective services and/or law enforcement; this may result in adolescents presenting with behaviors along a continuum from hostile to withdrawn.[9,11] Involved youth may withhold information or provide false information because they are protective of their exploiters, who are perceived as friends or romantic partners. It is also possible that youth involved in DMST may not provide an accurate history because of fear of their traffickers, attempting to avoid stigmatization of being labeled and/or formally charged as a prostitute, and dread of returning to a dysfunctional home living environment.[3,11]

When obtaining a medical history and completing an assessment, medical providers should be aware of the influence of patients' exploiters. It is important that providers are mindful that the recruiter/trafficker may be present with the patient during medical visits. Often a same-age peer accompanying a patient may be a recruiter, referred to as the bottom; a female appointed by the exploiter to supervise and report rule violations.[4,6] The involved youth may have been instructed to lie or not provide full information. Moreover, vulnerable minors may be psychologically controlled to the point that they remain under the influence of the exploiter and continue to comply with an exploiter's rules even when the exploiter is not physically present (eg, incarcerated).[9]

Provider Lack of Education/Awareness

The difficulties with identifying minors involved in DMST are compounded by clinicians' lack of experience, training, knowledge, and confidence regarding the identification of, medical management for, and resources available to victims of DMST survivors in the medical setting.[19,20] Study findings by Titchen and colleagues[19] revealed that although most medical trainees and physicians placed importance on knowing about human trafficking, they were unaware of the scope of the problem, what resources to seek, and appropriate interventions to provide trafficking survivors when they encountered them. Therefore, a standardized trafficking education curriculum for physicians, residents, and medical students is needed.

Signs of Involvement in Domestic Minor Sex Trafficking

To improve the identification of DMST involved youth, providers should be aware of potential physical, psychological, and medical indicators that are commonly associated with these vulnerable adolescents (**Table 1**).[3,11]

Table 1		
Potential indicators of domestic minor sex trafficking involvement		
Physical	**Psychological**	**Medical**
• Visible signs of abuse • Dressed in inappropriate clothing • Change in physical appearance over time • Reluctant to explain a certain tattoo • Unable to explain possession of expensive items	• Unexplained or multiple absences from home, school, or group home (may be hours to weeks) • Controlling relationships • Self-injurious behaviors • Suicidal ideation • Substance abuse	• History of multiple STIs • Multiple pregnancies (and possibly terminations) • Multiple sexual/physical assaults

Screening Questions

The presence of indicators does not definitively identify a patient as a DMST survivor, but may raise concern for the possibility of DMST. It is unclear whether all adolescents should be screened for DMST or only adolescents with 1 or more physical, psychological, and/or medial indicators, as described earlier. A uniform screening tool does not currently exist; however, the following questions were recommended by Greenbaum and Crawford-Jakubiak[3]:

1. Has anyone ever asked you to have sex in exchange for something you wanted or needed (money, food, shelter, or other items)?
2. Has anyone ever asked you to have sex with another person?
3. Has anyone ever taken sexual pictures of you or posted such pictures on the Internet?

Building rapport and reframing the screening questions to focus on a patient's friends, such as, "Have any of your friends been asked to have sex in exchange for something they wanted or needed?" may elicit additional information and sometimes more accurate information about the patient's own involvement.

MEDICAL RESPONSE
Acute Care

Involvement in DMST places the adolescent at risk for serious immediate and long-term physical and mental health consequences. These consequences include ongoing exposure to STIs, other infections (eg, skin infections from tattoos), traumatic injuries, substance abuse, pregnancy, mental health disorders (major depression, posttraumatic stress disorder, homicidality, and suicidality), poor compliance with general medical and dental care, or suboptimal care for previously identified medical problems (eg, asthma).[3,6,7,16]

Medical guidelines have been established by the American Academy of Pediatrics (AAP) and the American Professional Society on the Abuse of Children (APSAC) for patients who are victims of DMST, and these recommendations are based on existing guidelines for acute sexual assault patients.[3,7] It is important to use a trauma-informed approach for interviews and examinations of all possible DMST involved youth. A comprehensive examination with detailed documentation should include a thorough inspection for inflicted physical injury (eg, injuries inflicted by others, self-inflicted cutting, tattoos that may represent branding), sexual injury (acute and chronic anogenital trauma), malnutrition, and other neglect.[7] A genital examination, with the patient's consent, should be part of the medical examination to identify acute and chronic anogenital injuries (eg, lacerations, bleeding, abrasions, transections). A forensic evidence kit should also be offered if the last sexual encounter occurred within 72 hours of presentation for medical care, and has a likelihood for transfer of bodily fluids (blood, saliva, semen) based on the type of sexual contact reported.[3,7]

Patients should be tested for substance use/alcohol use, hepatitis, pregnancy, syphilis, chlamydia, gonorrhea, *Trichomonas*, and human immunodeficiency virus (HIV). Providers should follow the 2015 Centers for Disease Control and Prevention (CDC) STD guidelines for sexual abuse/assault patients.[21] Given the high probability of poor compliance with follow-up medical visits, it is generally advisable to provide prophylaxis for pregnancy and common STIs, including chlamydia, gonorrhea, and *Trichomonas* for DMST involved youth at the time of the initial evaluation.[7] The provision of HIV prophylaxis should be evaluated on a case-by-case basis. Medical providers should complete a risk assessment and communicate openly with the patient about their likelihood of adherence to the medication and follow-up visits. Consulting an infectious disease specialist and/or child abuse pediatrician is advisable to assist in making the determination regarding HIV prophylaxis.

During the acute medical visit, assess and treat acute and chronic medical and mental health conditions and provide referrals to appropriate community resources. It is important that providers are mindful of their obligation to meet mandatory reporting requirements to both child protective services and law enforcement because this varies from state to state. All states have mandatory reporting laws for child maltreatment. Many existing laws include the reporting of sex trafficking because it is a form of sexual exploitation. However, some state laws explicitly restrict reporting of child maltreatment to cases involving a parent, caregiver, or family member. Therefore, in some states sex trafficking does not meet the mandatory reporting requirement because the perpetrator is often not a parent or caregiver. Consulting a child abuse pediatrician and/or social workers may assist the provider with this decision.[22]

Follow-up Care

As is true for all adolescents, establishing a medical home for DMST survivors is essential.[23] Unique to the DMST patient population is the increased frequency of child protective services and/or law enforcement investigations caused by continued engagement in high-risk behaviors (eg, running away from home, multiple unprotected sexual encounters) that require additional medical evaluations. While identifying and treating emergent health issues during visits, medical providers should encourage the patient to comply with follow-up visits in order to adequately address ongoing medical and mental health care, repeat screening and testing for STIs, as well as safety planning.

Sexually Transmitted Infection Testing and Treatment

Follow-up testing and treatment of all STIs should be compliant with the 2015 CDC STD guidelines for sexual assault/abuse patients,[21] with the understanding that no specific guidelines exist for DMST patients. Thus, given the ongoing and high-risk exposures specific to this population, retesting beyond that stated in the CDC guidelines may be beneficial. Follow-up visits provide a crucial opportunity to detect new infections acquired during or after the initial evaluation and to monitor side effects and adherence to medications.

Pregnancy Prevention

The DMST population is at high risk for unplanned pregnancy. Patients should be offered emergency contraception when appropriate (See Ellen S. Rome and Veronica Issac's article, "Sometimes You Do Get a Second Chance: Emergency Contraception for Adolescents," in this issue). Birth control options should be reviewed with all adolescents, focusing on long-acting, reversible contraception (LARC) methods, which include injections, intrauterine devices (IUDs), and subdermal implants.[24] Despite past concerns, IUDs do not increase rates of STIs or pelvic inflammatory disease and therefore can be used in this population. LARC methods are viable options for DMST survivors to provide optimal pregnancy prevention given their transient living conditions, poor adherence to daily medications, and potential poor compliance with appointments for quarterly injections.[24]

Safety Planning

An important component of the medical response is establishing a safety plan, which must be prepared in concert with other professionals, such as law enforcement, child protective services, and community providers.[3] Safety planning evolves based on fluctuating circumstances of the patient and is similar to safety planning completed for IPV.

MULTIDISCIPLINARY RESPONSE

The provision of services to these survivors requires a coordinated, multisystem approach through the collaboration of child protective services; law enforcement (local, state, and federal); the office of the attorney general; social workers; educators; and mental health, medical, and other community providers.[3]

Many states have established specific DMST task forces to address legislative changes (safe harbor laws) and create a coordinated response once a survivor is encountered. Safe harbor laws provide immunity from prosecution and identify specific services for DMST involved youth. Safe harbor laws have been enacted in Connecticut, Florida, Illinois, Massachusetts, Minnesota, New York, Vermont, and Washington but vary from state to state.[11]

There remains a dearth of services and providers to address the multifaceted needs of these youth. The ultimate goal is to provide a safe environment for survivors to recover and establish a stable life outside of DMST.[11] Providers should be aware of established national resources available specifically for victimized and high-risk sex trafficked youth (**Box 1**).

Box 1
National resources for domestic minor sex trafficking survivors

- AAP Guidelines: http://pediatrics.aappublications.org/content/pediatrics/135/3/566.full.pdf
- APSAC Practice Guidelines: http://www.kyaap.org/wp-content/uploads/APSAC_Guidelines.pdf
- Girls Educational & Mentoring Services (GEMS): http://www.gems-girls.org
- Homeland Security: 1-(800) 973-2867
- Love 146: https://love146.org
- My Life My Choice: http://www.fightingexploitation.org
- National Human Trafficking Resource Center (NHTRC) hotline: 1-(888)-373-7888, http://traffickingresourcecenter.org
- The National Center for Missing and Exploited Children: 1-(800)-843-5678, http://www.missingkids.org/home

FUTURE DIRECTIONS

Although DMST has become an increasingly recognized issue, there is still a lot of work to be done in the domains of preventive efforts, identification, screening, appropriate interventions, and subsequent resource provision for victimized and high-risk youth. Adolescents involved in or at risk for DMST present frequently for medical attention and have recurrent interactions with health care providers[25]; thus, targeting DMST education, training, and research specifically in the medical setting is of paramount importance.

Standardized national medical protocols for DMST youth are needed to improve prevention, identification, and effective interventions (medical and social service provisions). Research should include a needs assessment of the knowledge gaps, barriers to screening, and performance on medical decision making of medical providers to inform future guidelines addressing acute and follow-up medical care.

With greater knowledge and awareness of DMST, medical institutions will have an improved opportunity to establish prevention efforts for both involved and at-risk youth, develop systematic strategies for identification and awareness of DMST, and establish community partnerships and referrals for intervention and safety planning.

REFERENCES

1. Victims of Trafficking and Violence Protection Act. Available at: http://www.state.gov/j/tip/laws/61124.htm. Accessed June 24, 2016.
2. United Nations Office on Drugs and Crime. Global report on trafficking in persons. Vienna (Austria): UNODC; 2014. Available at: htps://www.unodc.org/documents/data-and-analysis/glotip/GLOTIP_2014_full_report.pdf.
3. Greenbaum J, Crawford-Jakubiak JE, Committee on Child Abuse and Neglect. Child sex trafficking and commercial sexual exploitation: health care needs of victims. Pediatrics 2015;135(3):566–74.
4. The polaris project. Myths & misconceptions. National Human Trafficking Resource Center. Office on trafficking in Persons. Administration for Children and Families. U.S. Department of Health and Human Services (HHS); 2014. Available at: https://traffickingresourcecenter.org/what-human-trafficking/myths-misconceptions. Accessed August 23, 2016.
5. Edwards JM, Iritani BJ, Hallfors DD. Prevalence and correlates of exchanging sex for drugs or money among adolescents in the United States. Sex Transm Infect 2006;82(5):354–8.
6. Estes R, Weiner N. The commercial sexual exploitation of children in the U.S., Canada and Mexico. Philadelphia: Center for the Study of Youth Policy, University of Pennsylvania; 2001.
7. American Professional Society on the Abuse of Children. The commercial sexual exploitation of children: the medical provider's role in identification, assessment and treatment: APSAC practice guidelines. Chicago: APSAC; 2013. Available at: www.kyaap.org/wp-content/uploads/APSAC_Guidelines.pdf. Accessed March 30, 2016.
8. Muftic LR, Finn MA. Health outcomes among women trafficked for sex in the United States: a closer look. J Interpers Violence 2013;28(9):1859–85.
9. Smith LA, Vardaman SH, Snow MA. Domestic minor sex trafficking. Available at: http://sharedhope.org/wp-content/uploads/2012/09/SHI_National_ Report_on_DMST_2009.pdf. Accessed December 11, 2015.
10. Hazen E, Schlozman S, Beresin E. Adolescent psychological development. Pediatr Rev 2008;29(5):161–7.

11. Institute of Medicine and National Research Council. Confronting commercial sexual exploitation and sex trafficking of minors in the United States. Washington, DC: The National Academies Press; 2013.
12. Clawson HJ, Dutch N, Solomon A, et al. Human trafficking into and within the United States: a review of the literature. Study of HHS Programs Serving Human Trafficking Victims. Available at: http://aspe.hhs.gov/hsp/07/HumanTrafficking/LitRev/. Accessed January 5, 2016.
13. Jenny C, editor. Child abuse and neglect: diagnosis, treatment, and evidence. St Louis (MO): Saunders, Elsevier; 2011.
14. Raphael J, Reichert JA, Powers M, et al. Pimp control and violence: domestic sex trafficking of Chicago women and girls. Women Crim Justice 2010;20(1–2): 89–104.
15. Kennedy MA, Klein C, Bristowe JT, et al. Pimps' techniques and other circumstances that lead to street prostitution. Journal of Aggression, Maltreatment & Trauma 2007;15(2):1–19.
16. Curtis R, Terry K, Dank M, et al. The commercial sexual exploitation of children in New York city: Volume 1: The CSEC population in New York city: size, characteristics, and needs [Internet]. Washington, DC: National Institute of Justice, US Department of Justice; 2008. Available at: www.ncjrs.gov/pdffiles1/nij/grants/ 225083.pdf. Accessed October 2, 2015.
17. Pence E, Paymar M. Education groups for men who batter. New York: Springer Publishing Company; 1993.
18. Adams W, Owens C, Small K. Effects of federal legislation on the commercial exploitation of children. Rockville (MD): Office of Juvenile Justice and Delinquency Prevention; 2010. Available at: https://www.ncjrs.gov/pdffiles1/ojjdp/ 228631.pdf. Accessed August 22, 2016.
19. Titchen KE, Loo D, Berdan E, et al. Domestic sex trafficking of minors: medical student and physician awareness. J Pediatr Adolesc Gynecol 2015;30(1):102–8.
20. Beck M, Lineer M, Melzer-Lange M, et al. Medical providers' understanding of sex trafficking and their experience with at-risk patients. Pediatrics 2015;135(4): e895–902.
21. Centers for Disease Control and Prevention. Sexual Assault and Abuse and STDs. 2015. Available at: https://www.cdc.gov/std/tg2015/sexual-assault.htm# pep. Accessed June 5, 2016.
22. Atkinson HG, Curnin KJ, Hanson NC. U.S. state laws addressing human trafficking: education of and mandatory reporting by health care providers and other professionals. Journal of Human Trafficking 2016;2(2):111–38.
23. Medical Home Initiatives for Children with Special Needs Project Advisory Committee, American Academy of Pediatrics. The medical home. Pediatrics 2002; 110(1):184–6.
24. Ott MA, Sucato GS. Committee on adolescents. Contraception for adolescents. Pediatrics 2014;134(4):e1257–81.
25. Lederer L, Wetzel CA. The health consequences of sex trafficking and their implications for identifying victims in health care facilities. Ann Health Law 2014;23: 61–91.

Prevention of and Interventions for Dating and Sexual Violence in Adolescence

Elizabeth Miller, MD, PhD

KEYWORDS

- Dating violence • Sexual violence • Adolescence • Violence prevention
- Relationship abuse

KEY POINTS

- Dating violence (also known as adolescent relationship abuse) and sexual violence are prevalent from the middle school years throughout adolescence and peak in young adulthood.
- Dating and sexual violence victimization are associated with multiple poor physical and mental health consequences, including unintended pregnancy and sexually transmitted infections.
- Health care providers can promote healthy adolescent sexual relationships by offering universal education and brief anticipatory guidance with all adolescent patients about healthy and unhealthy relationships and sexual consent.

BACKGROUND

Prevalence of Adolescent Relationship Abuse and Sexual Violence

Adolescence is a critical developmental period for exploring sexual and gender identity, sexual attractions, relationships, dating, and intimacy. The middle school years represent a particularly critical stage for relationship abuse and sexual violence education and prevention, as many youth start establishing romantic or sexual relationships for the first time.[1,2] Sexual harassment increases during middle school,[3–6] with studies identifying such experiences as early as sixth grade and persisting into high school.[7–10] Increased interactions with the opposite sex during the middle school years correlate with increasing rates of opposite-sex aggressive encounters in middle school.[4] Even though younger adolescents have less experience with formal dating relationships, early gender-based conflicts do occur.[1,11] Advances in brain development science

Disclosure Statement: The author has nothing to disclose.
Division of Adolescent and Young Adult Medicine, Pediatrics, Children's Hospital of Pittsburgh of UPMC, University of Pittsburgh School of Medicine, 3420 Fifth Avenue, Pittsburgh, PA 15213, USA
E-mail address: elizabeth.miller@chp.edu

indicate that the highly dynamic pubertal transition (the hallmark of middle school years) is a period of intense social emotional learning, changes in thought regulation and reasoning, and empathy maturity.[12] For most tweens and young teens, new peer and social influences come into play, and pressure to conform may be felt in powerful ways. This may be the first time behaviors they have seen in their families, and lessons learned from peers and popular culture, manifest in their own relationships. Health care providers play a key role in providing anticipatory guidance to their patients in early adolescence regarding the importance of healthy romantic and sexual relationships.

Teen dating violence (herein referred to as adolescent relationship abuse [ARA]) denotes the emotional, physical, or sexual abuse of a dating or sexual partner. The abuse can take place in person, online or via texting, or through a third party (eg, a peer conveying a message or threat). Abusive and controlling behaviors may take the form of monitoring a partner's cell phone use, telling partners what they can wear, controlling where and with whom they hang out, manipulating contraceptive use, and other possessive behaviors. The term "adolescent relationship abuse," rather than "teen dating violence," helps to emphasize that abusive and controlling behaviors can occur in early adolescence (before teen years) and extend into young adulthood (the highest prevalence of partner violence is among young adults ages 18–24), spanning all of adolescence. The term "abuse" helps underscore that many abusive behaviors are neither physical nor violent. Similarly, adolescents use many terms (not only "dating") to refer to their sexual and intimate relationships.

Nationwide, approximately 1 in 10 high school students has been hit, slapped, or physically hurt on purpose by a boyfriend or girlfriend. Sexual violence is also common in the context of ARA. The most recent national Youth Risk Behavior Surveillance System survey findings of high school students included a question about sexual violence victimization in the context of a dating relationship with 14% of adolescent girls and 6% of adolescent boys reporting such violence in the past year.[13] Sexual violence (SV) (including sexual coercion, nonconsensual sexual contact, and rape) is common, with 28% to 56% of women in college samples reporting at least 1 such experience.[14,15] More than three-quarters of women who have been sexually assaulted report that the first of such experiences occurred before the age of 25, underscoring that partner and sexual violence are adolescent and young adult concerns.[16]

Unique characteristics of adolescent relationship abuse

Depending on the adolescent's stage of social/emotional development, the young person may not recognize the warning signs of abuse, confusing the controlling behaviors and possessiveness as signs of "true love." Similarly, a young person may defer seeking care due to multiple barriers, including fear of breaches of confidentiality, lack of trust in adult providers, a desire to protect the abusive partner, self-blame, and inability to access care. The health care provider should always consider the adolescent's developmental stage, and discuss concrete and specific behaviors ("does she or he get mad at you if you don't respond to his or her calls right away?") rather than vague questions, such as "Are you in an abusive relationship?" In addition, in some communities, adolescents use different terms to describe ARA.[17] Knowledge of and/or clarifying the use of local terms for relationships can create a shared understanding of what behaviors constitute ARA and may help initiate the discussion of ARA.

Reproductive coercion

ARA is associated with increased sexual risk behavior and sexually transmitted infections (STIs).[18] ARA also has been associated with teen pregnancy, with up to two-thirds of such pregnancies occurring in the context of an abusive relationship. Unintended pregnancies, which make up more than 80% of adolescent pregnancies, are also 2 to 3 times more likely to be associated with abuse than intended pregnancies at any time during the 12 months before conception or during pregnancy. Condom nonuse,[19] inconsistent condom use,[19,20] and fear of condom negotiation[19] are common among abused adolescents. Lack of control over contraception, coupled with coercive or forced unprotected sex, is a recognized mechanism in elevating risk for unintended pregnancy, as well as human immunodeficiency virus (HIV) and other STIs for both boys and girls.[21,22]

Evidence in the past decade has identified reproductive coercion (ie, partner pressure to get pregnant, condom manipulation, and birth control sabotage) as an additional mechanism for increasing a young woman's risk for unintended pregnancy.[22–26] In a study among young women using family planning clinics, 25% had ever experienced reproductive coercion, which was associated with unintended pregnancy.[24] Reproductive coercion is more likely to occur in the context of ARA, yet adolescent girls may not recognize these behaviors as abusive or detrimental to their health. Adolescents and young adult women who are seeking care for STI testing, pregnancy testing, and requesting emergency contraception are also more likely to be experiencing ARA and reproductive coercion.[27] Health care providers may need to inquire directly about reproductive coercion. Discussion with adolescent patients about ARA and reproductive coercion may facilitate adolescent recognition of ARA and encourage use of harm-reduction behaviors to increase safety and reduce risk for STI and pregnancy.

Cyber dating abuse

Texting, social networking sites, and cell phones are ubiquitous. This electronic networking, although building positive social connections, can become an arena for exploitation and abuse, including excessive texting, "sexting" (transmitting nude images of oneself or one's partner), spying, or constant cell phone monitoring. Emerging research among adolescents has highlighted the prevalence of cyber dating abuse (use of technology to control or harass a partner),[28,29] which is also associated with poor reproductive and sexual health outcomes. In a study with students seeking care in School-Based Health Centers (SBHCs) in northern California, lifetime prevalence of physical or sexual ARA victimization was 25%, with 13% reporting such abuse in the past 3 months.[30] Recent cyber dating abuse was reported by 41% of this clinic sample. Among female participants, even low levels of cyber dating abuse exposure was associated with lower rates of contraceptive use (adjusted odds ratio [AOR] 1.8, 95% confidence interval [CI] 1.2–2.7) and more reproductive coercion (AOR 3.0, 95% CI 1.4–6.2), underscoring the association of relationship abuse (including cyber abuse) with pregnancy risk.[28] Health care providers should include discussion of the benefits, as well as risks, associated with social media with young patients and their parents, including how to set limits and maintain privacy (see www.thatsnotcool.com for teens to learn about setting their own "digital line").

Sexual and Reproductive Health Impacts

ARA (including reproductive coercion and cyber dating abuse) and SV are associated with many poor health outcomes[18,24,31,32]:

- Unintended pregnancy
- STIs including HIV
- Injuries

- Poor academic performance
- Depression and suicidality
- Substance abuse
- Disordered eating

ARA is prevalent among adolescents seeking care in confidential settings, such as family planning and SBHCs, with lifetime estimates ranging from 40% to 53%, significantly higher than national estimates in the general adolescent population (approximately 20% of adolescent girls and 10% of boys),[13,33,34] and more than 25% of teens seeking clinical care reporting physical and SV from a partner and 40% reporting cyber dating abuse.[28,30] Given the many negative physical and mental health consequences of ARA, adolescents may be seeking clinical services for conditions associated with ARA, yet may not recognize or disclose that they are in an abusive or unhealthy relationship. Health professionals have a critical role in providing universal education and anticipatory guidance for all adolescent patients.

Preparing Your Practice

In comparison to adult domestic violence, ARA involves at least one minor. The health care provider is required to balance the safety of the minor while creating safe spaces that are confidential for adolescents to share experiences with their provider. Providers need to know their state's minor consent/confidentiality and mandated reporting requirements for child abuse, neglect, and sexual abuse. Before providing universal education about healthy and unhealthy relationships, health care providers should disclose the limits of confidentiality to their adolescent patients.

> I am so glad you are here today. Before we get started, I want to remind you that I value your privacy. That said, I also want to make sure you know that there are various laws in this state to help keep young people safe. So if I have a young person in clinic who is going to hurt herself or himself or someone is hurting them, I sometimes have to get other adults involved to help keep them safe. What questions do you have about that?

Knowledge of these reporting requirements and how to support an adolescent in the safest way possible requires consultation. Developing connections with colleagues (eg, social workers, domestic violence agencies, rape crisis centers) to discuss options and reporting requirements is essential. Reporting a case to an outside agency without carefully considering safety could place the young person at significantly greater risk for harm.

Assessment for Relationship Abuse and Sexual Violence

Given the prevalence of ARA, including cyber dating abuse and reproductive coercion in adolescent clinical settings, interventions designed to reduce ARA may promote healthier sexual decision making and reduce risk for STI and unintended pregnancies.

Primary prevention

Talk with all adolescent patients about the importance of healthy relationships (including sexual communication) and provide information on supports and resources related to ARA and SV that they can share with friends.

Early intervention

Connect youth experiencing ARA and SV to appropriate trauma-focused counseling and advocacy services, as in the following example.

Universal education around healthy relationships normalizes and contextualizes inquiry about ARA:

I talk to all of my patients about the importance of healthy relationships, how everyone deserves to be treated with trust and respect. Some of my patients tell me about how the people they're seeing are constantly checking up on them or putting them down, has anything like that happened to you?

And when the young person says, "No" to the question, follow-up with sharing an educational resource (see for example, a palm-sized educational brochure described later in this article and available at https://www.futureswithoutviolence.org/hanging-out-or-hooking-up-teen-safety-card/):

I'm glad to hear that's not happening to you. You might have a friend who can use this information. If you're interested, please take this along with you. You can take 2 or 3 to share.

It is not unusual for adolescents to disclose that they are victims of ARA to their friends rather than to their parents or other adults. This enables providers to raise the topic of ARA as it pertains to the patient's peer group, not just to the individual. This approach of offering information "to help a friend" also reduces the stigma for a young person, so she or he does not feel as if the provider is focusing only on her/him.

We make sure to talk about unhealthy relationships with all of our patients, because you may know someone for whom this information might be useful. Please know that this is a safe place to bring friends you are concerned about.

Experiences of abuse and violence cluster with other common adolescent health and social problems. Adolescents experiencing violence in their homes from adult caregivers are more likely to experience abusive relationships with a partner. In an attempt to leave the abusive family living situation, they may seek out a less-monitored peer setting, and thus become more vulnerable to unhealthy, abusive, or exploitative relationships. Adolescents experiencing ARA are also more likely to be depressed, use substances, and engage in unprotected intercourse (increasing risk for pregnancy and infections). This means that when addressing any other adolescent behavior relevant to a young person's health and well-being (whether it is smoking, school performance, unprotected sex, substance use, or nonsuicidal self-injury), the provider should *consider the possibility of an abusive relationship as part of the differential diagnosis.*

With a young person who has had several STIs, a provider might say, *"When I see a pattern of infections like this, I worry about someone making you do things sexual that you did not want to do. Could that be part of your story?"*

And regardless of whether the young person discloses an abusive relationship or not, the provider should always offer ARA-related information. *"We're giving this information to all our patients, as we really care that our patients are in healthy relationships."*

Clinical red flags
In addition to universal discussions about ARA with patients, providers should be alert to particular signs and symptoms that may signal the possibility that a patient is using abuse in a relationship, being abused, or both. Adolescents may present with nonspecific complaints, such as recurrent headaches, poor sleep, abdominal pain, or fatigue. Depression, anxiety, disordered eating, suicidal ideation, and substance misuse all

co-occur with ARA and SV exposure. Frequent requests for pregnancy testing, STI testing, and use of emergency contraception are also associated with ARA.

In the presence of such "clinical red flags," providers should conduct a more thorough assessment, providing education on what constitutes abusive behavior (regardless of whether the young person discloses an abusive relationship or not), offering harm-reduction strategies that may help a young person reduce their risk for abuse and violence, as well as ensuring that the young person is aware of specific resources and supports in the community to support victims of violence.

For example, for an adolescent who has been diagnosed with an STI, such as Chlamydia, notifying her sexual partner about the need to be treated for an infection can be challenging, and even more so in the context of an abusive relationship. Providers can assess for safety by inquiring, *"How is the person you are having sex with going to react when they hear that they need to be treated, too?"* To help adolescent patients stay safer (harm reduction), providers can offer to speak with the partner and offer treatment, assist the patient in using an anonymous Web site to notify sex partners (such as www.sotheycanknow.org), or contact the partner anonymously by phone.

Universal education, brief counseling, and warm referrals

There are several reasons why best practice is to provide *universal education and brief counseling to all patients about ARA*, rather than relying on a survey or checklist and simply screening youth for violence exposure and responding only to disclosures.

First, a primary prevention approach may be more feasible and more effective in the context of primary care. Raising the topic of ARA and SV with patients with the explicit goal of having them disseminate the information to peers, or becoming "positive upstanders" (rather than passive and silent bystanders) in peer ARA situations, can reduce ARA in the population. Perceived peer approval of ARA and associated SV contributes to attitudes sanctioning such behavior. Engaging youth as active bystanders in preventing ARA and SV is one strategy for promoting change within social contexts.[35] Additionally, conveying ARA education by encouraging youth to be prepared to help a friend facilitates both provision and receipt of this sensitive information that reduces stigma and promotes more positive bystander behavior.

Second, universal education is important because not all youth recognize abusive behaviors as problematic. Providing information about healthy and unhealthy relationship behaviors may help youth remain vigilant when they meet new partners. The lack of recognition of abusive behaviors in relationships[36,37] has been associated with lower help-seeking for abuse,[38] highlighting need for education. Qualitative studies have indicated that survivors want health providers to be sensitive to how difficult it can be to disclose interpersonal violence to a health provider, and want information, resources, and support *regardless of disclosure*.[39] In one intervention trial, the practice of informing all female family planning patients about partner violence and reproductive coercion benefited all women; women who received the intervention, both those who were and were not experiencing abuse, were 63% more likely than those in the control group to end a relationship because they perceived the relationship to be unhealthy or unsafe.[40] A patient who checks "no" on a screening question or does not disclose exposure to violence during a clinical encounter may have a myriad reasons for nondisclosure, including not recognizing their experiences as abuse, feeling shame, and fearing the consequences of disclosure. Provision of ARA-relevant information to all patients reduces the stigma around violence exposure, educates youth about what they deserve in a relationship, and communicates that the clinic is a safe space for talking about relationship concerns.

Third, providing brief counseling about steps a young person might take to protect herself from specific harms that occur in the context of ARA can make an important difference. Harm reduction is effective in managing a range of health risk behaviors,[41] including sexual health[42–44] and partner violence.[45] A goal of the universal education approach is to provide examples of harm-reduction strategies that adolescents can use for themselves or their peers; examples include how to reduce their risk for ARA victimization and sexual risk via contraceptive options that do not require partner knowledge, safer strategies for STI partner notification (example offered previously), safer condom negotiation, reducing isolation, connecting with safe adults, and breaking up safely. A recent trial in family planning clinics found that all clients who received the universal education and brief counseling about harm-reduction strategies had significant increases in knowledge of available resources and in self-efficacy to enact harm-reduction behaviors.[40]

Finally, the universal education approach creates an opportunity to share with adolescent patients that there are adults in health care who are able to provide support and guidance to young people exposed to ARA or SV. The trust and rapport that the health care provider has with an adolescent patient can serve as a "bridge" to advocacy services and counseling as appropriate. A warm referral is the process of connecting a patient directly with an advocate (in person, or by phone or telemedicine) rather than simply providing a number to call. Making warm referrals to victim service advocates can assist clients in overcoming barriers to accessing services, including self-blame,[37,46] lack of recognition of abuse,[38] lack of knowledge of services,[37,46,47] and perception that services are limited in scope (eg, solely crisis oriented).[46] Describing the scope of services available and normalizing use of such services may facilitate awareness and use of ARA services, improve mental health symptoms,[48–50] and reduce re-victimization.[51] Providers can benefit from establishing formal agreements and connections with local violence-related services relevant for adolescents to communicate the availability of these teen-friendly ARA resources and to support adolescents in making the connection to these resources when appropriate. This may include allowing a young person to use the phone in clinic to call and speak with an advocate (rather than using her own cell phone) or setting up a time that an advocate can come meet with the young person in clinic.

Creating a safe environment for possible disclosure
A supportive and safe environment includes having posters, brochures, and messages in the clinical space about relationships and love that are geared toward adolescents. Brochures that provide education about ARA lay the groundwork for a conversation with the provider. The materials used should be multicultural, depict same-sex and opposite-sex relationships, and avoid "victim-blaming" language (see www.love isrespoot.org and www.futureswithioutviolence.org for teen relevant materials).

Framing the conversation
Every encounter with an adolescent in the health care setting is an opportunity to educate youth about what healthy relationships are, the ways in which unhealthy relationships affect their health, and how health care providers are prepared to support youth experiencing abuse and violence in their relationships. Although it may seem counterintuitive, the goal is *not* to extract a disclosure from the young person, because it is not essential that the provider knows whether or not the patient has experienced abuse to provide helpful information and motivate the patient to take action on his or her own to improve safety. The goal is to ensure that patients leave clinic with information about ARA-relevant resources, that they know the clinic is a safe place to

discuss such concerns, and that they know the provider is comfortable with discussing sensitive topics and can be an important ally for them.

Universalizing *Many of our patients have shared with us how they have experienced situations in their relationships that made them feel uncomfortable and even scared. We care about this a lot as health care providers, because unhealthy relationships can really affect your health. We now talk to all of our patients about their relationships because you and your health are really important to us.*

Educational *Because relationships can have such an impact on the health of young people, we have been sharing this information with all of our patients, because it is likely you know someone who could use this information. We want you to know that this is a safe place for young people to share with us the issues that they are concerned about. [share educational card]*

Concrete *Does this person ever tell you where you can go or who you can talk to?*

Do they need to know where you are all the time? Do they check your cell phone to see everyone you have called?

Do they ever try to make you have sex when you don't want to?

Do they ever totally lose it, throw things?

Collaborative model for care

Given the complexities of caring for adolescents, providers should identify the resources in their community where there are specialists in partner and SV. These individuals and/or agencies are helpful for consultation and referral.

- Identify a local domestic violence agency and/or rape crisis center and invite staff from those agencies to attend meetings with clinic staff. Have materials from the agency readily available in examination rooms and know how to reach an advocate (if geographically close, some advocates may even come to the clinic to meet with a patient).
- Connect with allies in mental health, social work, behavioral pediatrics, and adolescent medicine, as well as other local community resources, such as domestic violence and rape crisis centers, child protection services, and legal advocates familiar with youth law.
- Create an adolescent-friendly environment in the clinical setting, and enlist other clinic staff in helping to create a "safe" space for teens that conveys respect for youth strengths, privacy, and self-determination.
- Ensure that all youth in the practice receive information on relationship abuse, SV, and healthy relationships. These materials should resonate with them regardless of gender and sexual identity. Adolescents should leave the clinic knowing that the clinic team cares about them, their relationships, and their well-being.

Example of universal education and brief counseling intervention

The Healthcare Education Assessment and Response for Teen Relationships intervention (HEART) is a provider-delivered universal education and brief counseling intervention for boys and girls seeking routine care that has been tested in SBHCs (comprehensive health centers located in high schools). In a cluster randomized controlled trial, youth seeking services at intervention SBHCs were more likely to report increased knowledge of ARA resources, increased self-efficacy to use harm-reduction strategies, increased disclosure of ARA during their clinic visit, and less ARA victimization 3 months later.[30]

The HEART intervention is universal, inclusive of all gender and sexual identities and clinic visit types, addressing a range of abusive behaviors, including cyber dating abuse and reproductive coercion. The *core intervention components* are as follows:

1. SBHC provider–delivered ARA information and resources regardless of disclosure (universal education)

2. ARA assessment including for reproductive and sexual coercion and discussion of harm-reduction strategies to reduce risk for ARA and sexual risk

3. Supported referrals to victim service advocates (referrals made via phone or in person during the clinic visit)

4. Peer-to-peer sharing of information to raise awareness about ARA and availability of the SBHC for support; all SBHC users receive a card with ARA information.

Partnering with schools and youth serving agencies on prevention of adolescent relationship abuse and sexual violence

Health care providers serving adolescents and young adults may also want to partner with community-based agencies and schools to ensure greater dissemination of evidence-based ARA and SV prevention programs.

Examples of evidence-based prevention programs for use in schools include:

- Shifting Boundaries: a middle school classroom and school environment SV prevention intervention (http://www.nij.gov/topics/crime/intimate-partner-violence/teen-dating-violence/documents/shifting-boundaries-all-schools.pdf)
- Fourth R: a high school student classroom-based curriculum on healthy youth relationships (https://youthrelationships.org/)
- Green Dot: a high school and college campus bystander intervention program (https://www.livethegreendot.com/)
- Coaching Boys into Men: athletic coaches (middle school or high school) deliver weekly messages to their athletes about stopping violence against women and girls (http://www.coachescorner.org/)

Sexual exploitation of minors

ARA sometimes co-occurs with other forms of violence victimization, including parent-to-child abuse or neglect, bullying, sexual abuse, or commercial sexual exploitation. Although beyond the scope of this article, adolescents experiencing relationship abuse may be especially vulnerable to sexual exploitation (see Jessica L. Moore and colleagues' article, "Sex Trafficking of Minors," in this issue). The national hotline for human trafficking victimization can be used for advice and consultation: (888) 373-7888.

REFERENCES

1. Noonan RK, Charles D. Developing teen dating violence prevention strategies formative research with middle school youth. Violence Against Women 2009; 15(9):1087–105.
2. Stein N. Sexual harassment in school—the public performance of gendered violence. Harv Educ Rev 1995;65(2):145–62.
3. McMaster LE, Connolly J, Pepler D, et al. Peer to peer sexual harassment in early adolescence: a developmental perspective. Dev Psychopathol 2002;14(1): 91–105.

4. Pellegrini AD. A longitudinal study of heterosexual relationships, aggression, and sexual harassment during the transition from primary school through middle school. J Appl Dev Psychol 2001;22(2):119–33.

5. Bentley CG, Galliher RV, Ferguson TJ. Associations among aspects of interpersonal power and relationship functioning in adolescent romantic couples. Sex Roles 2007;57(7–8):483–95.

6. Manganello JA. Teens, dating violence, and media use—a review of the literature and conceptual model for future research. Trauma Violence Abuse 2008;9(1): 3–18.

7. Taylor BG, Stein ND, Mumford EA, et al. Shifting Boundaries: an experimental evaluation of a dating violence prevention program in middle schools. Prev Sci 2013;14(1):64–76.

8. O'Keefe M. Predictors of dating violence among high school students. J Interpers Violence 1997;12(4):546–68.

9. Callahan MR, Tolman RM, Saunders DG. Adolescent dating violence victimization and psychological well-being. J Adolesc Res 2003;18(6):664–81.

10. Eaton DK, Kann L, Kinchen S, et al. Youth risk behavior surveillance—United States, 2009. MMWR Surveill Summ 2010;59(5):1–142.

11. Mulford C, Giordano PC. Teen dating violence: a closer look at adolescent romantic relationships. Washington, DC: National Institute of Justice; 2008. p. 261.

12. Baird AA, Fugelsang JA. The emergence of consequential thought: evidence from neuroscience. Philos Trans R Soc Lond B Biol Sci 2004;359(1451): 1791–804.

13. Vagi KJ, O'Malley Olsen E, Basile KC, et al. Teen dating violence (physical and sexual) among US high school students: findings from the 2013 National Youth Risk Behavior Survey. JAMA Pediatr 2015;169(5):474–82.

14. Mouilso ER, Fischer S, Calhoun KS. A prospective study of sexual assault and alcohol use among first-year college women. Violence Vict 2012;27(1):78–94.

15. Johnson NL, Johnson DM. Factors influencing the relationship between sexual trauma and risky sexual behavior in college students. J Interpers Violence 2013;28(11):2315–31.

16. Black M, Basile K, Breiding M, et al. The National Intimate Partner and Sexual Violence Survey (NISVS): 2010 summary report. Atlanta (GA): National Center for Injury Prevention and Control Centers for Disease Control and Prevention; 2011.

17. Martin CE, Houston AM, Mmari KN, et al. Urban teens and young adults describe drama, disrespect, dating violence and help-seeking preferences. Matern Child Health J 2012;16(5):957–66.

18. Decker MR, Silverman JG, Raj A. Dating violence and sexually transmitted disease/HIV testing and diagnosis among adolescent females. Pediatrics 2005; 116(2):e272–6.

19. Sales JM, Salazar LF, Wingood GM, et al. The mediating role of partner communication skills on HIV/STD-associated risk behaviors in young African American females with a history of sexual violence. Arch Pediatr Adolesc Med 2008; 162(5):432–8.

20. Teitelman AM, Ratcliffe SJ, Morales-Aleman MM, et al. Sexual relationship power, intimate partner violence, and condom use among minority urban girls. J Interpers Violence 2008;23(12):1694–712.

21. McFarlane J, Malecha A, Watson K, et al. Intimate partner sexual assault against women: frequency, health consequences, and treatment outcomes. Obstet Gynecol 2005;105(1):99–108.
22. Miller E, Silverman J. Reproductive coercion and partner violence: implications for clinical assessment of unintended pregnancy. Expert Rev Obstet Gynecol 2010;5(5):511–5.
23. Miller E, McCauley HL, Tancredi DJ, et al. Recent reproductive coercion and unintended pregnancy among female family planning clients. Contraception 2014; 89(2):122–8.
24. Miller E, Decker MR, McCauley HL, et al. Pregnancy coercion, intimate partner violence, and uinintended pregnancy. Contraception 2010;81(4):316–22.
25. Miller E, Decker MR, Reed E, et al. Male pregnancy promoting behaviors and adolescent partner violence: findings from a qualitative study with adolescent females. Ambul Pediatr 2007;7(5):360–6.
26. Moore AM, Frohwirth L, Miller E. Male reproductive control of women who have experienced intimate partner violence in the United States. Soc Sci Med 2010; 70(11):1737–44.
27. Kazmerski T, McCauley HL, Jones K, et al. Use of reproductive and sexual health services among female family planning clinic clients exposed to partner violence and reproductive coercion. Matern Child Health J 2015;19(7):1490–6.
28. Dick RN, McCauley HL, Jones KA, et al. Cyber dating abuse among teens using school-based health centers. Pediatrics 2014;134(6):e1560–7.
29. Zweig JM, Dank M, Yahner J, et al. The rate of cyber dating abuse among teens and how it relates to other forms of teen dating violence. J Youth Adolesc 2013; 42(7):1063–77.
30. Miller E, Goldstein S, McCauley HL, et al. A school health center intervention for abusive adolescent relationships: a cluster RCT. Pediatrics 2015;135(1):76–85.
31. Exner-Cortens D, Eckenrode J, Rothman E. Longitudinal associations between teen dating violence victimization and adverse health outcomes. Pediatrics 2013;131(1):71–8.
32. Foshee V, Reyes H, Gottfredson N, et al. A longitudinal examination of psychological, behavioral, academic, and relationship consequences of dating abuse victimization among a primarily rural sample of adolescents. J Adolesc Health 2013;53(6):723–9.
33. Miller E, Decker M, Raj A, et al. Intimate partner violence and health care-seeking patterns among female users of urban adolescent clinics. Matern Child Health J 2010;14(6):910–7.
34. Keeling J, Birch L. The prevalence rates of domestic abuse in women attending a family planning clinic. J Fam Plann Reprod Health Care 2004;30(2):113–4.
35. Banyard VL, Plante EG, Moynihan MM. Bystander education: bringing a broader community perspective to sexual violence prevention. J Community Psychol 2004;32(1):61–79.
36. Chang JC, Decker M, Moracco KE, et al. What happens when health care providers ask about intimate partner violence? A description of consequences from the perspectives of female survivors. J Am Med Womens Assoc 2003; 58(2):76–81.
37. Hathaway JE, Willis G, Zimmer B. Listening to survivors' voices: addressing partner abuse in the health care setting. Violence Against Women 2002;8(6):687–719.
38. Rickert VI, Wiemann CM, Vaughan RD. Disclosure of date/acquaintance rape: who reports and when. J Pediatr Adolesc Gynecol 2005;18(1):17–24.

39. Chang JC, Decker MR, Moracco KE, et al. Asking about intimate partner violence: advice from female survivors to health care providers. Patient Educ Couns 2005;59(2):141–7.
40. Miller E, Decker MR, McCauley HL, et al. A family planning clinic partner violence intervention to reduce risk associated with reproductive coercion. Contraception 2011;83(3):274–80.
41. Marlatt G. Harm reduction: pragmatic strategies for managing high risk behaviors. New York: Guilford Press; 1998.
42. Fry CL, Treloar C, Maher L. Ethical challenges and responses in harm reduction research: promoting applied communitarian ethics. Drug Alcohol Rev 2005;24(5): 449–59.
43. Gielen AC, McDonald EM, Wilson ME, et al. Effects of improved access to safety counseling, products, and home visits on parents' safety practices: results of a randomized trial. Arch Pediatr Adolesc Med 2002;156(1):33–40.
44. Heller D, McCoy K, Cunningham C. An invisible barrier to integrating HIV primary care with harm reduction services: philosophical clashes between the harm reduction and medical models. Public Health Rep 2004;119(1):32–9.
45. Kurtz S, Surratt HL, Inciardi JA, et al. Sex work and "date" violence. Violence Against Women 2004;10:357–85.
46. Logan TK, Evans L, Stevenson E, et al. Barriers to services for rural and urban survivors of rape. J Interpers Violence 2005;20(5):591–616.
47. Du Mont J, Forte T, Cohen MM, et al. Changing help-seeking rates for intimate partner violence in Canada. Women Health 2005;41(1):1–19.
48. Bennett L, Riger S, Schewe P, et al. Effectiveness of hotline, advocacy, counseling, and shelter services for victims of domestic violence: a statewide evaluation. J Interpers Violence 2004;19(7):815–29.
49. Starzynski LL, Ullman SE, Filipas HH, et al. Correlates of women's sexual assault disclosure to informal and formal support sources. Violence Vict 2005;20(4): 417–32.
50. Wasco SM, Campbell R, Howard A, et al. A statewide evaluation of services provided to rape survivors. J Interpers Violence 2004;19(2):252–63.
51. Sullivan CM, Bybee DI. Reducing violence using community-based advocacy for women with abusive partners. J Consult Clin Psychol 1999;67(1):43–53.

Sexuality and Disability in Adolescents

Cynthia Holland-Hall, MD, MPH[a],*, Elisabeth H. Quint, MD[b]

KEYWORDS

- Sexuality • Disability • Adolescent • Sexuality education

KEY POINTS

- Sexuality is a topic that may be neglected in adolescents with disabilities, despite evidence that their needs are often similar to or greater than those of their typically developing peers.
- Several hormonal treatment options are available to assist with menstrual management and provide contraception.
- Medical providers may facilitate healthy sexual development in adolescents with disabilities by initiating conversations with patients and caregivers about sexuality.

INTRODUCTION

When caring for adolescents, providers may feel ill equipped to address issues of sexuality. In part, this may reflect the tendency to equate "sexuality" with "sexual intercourse." Sexual development is a multidimensional process that spans childhood, adolescence, and adulthood. Young children explore gender expression, discover body parts, and learn to respect others' personal space. Children of all ages witness and process the sexual images and relationships seen in their environment. Adolescents undergo the changes of puberty, experience sexual feelings and desires, and develop the capacity for intimacy and reproduction. The process sometimes proves challenging for adolescents and their caregivers, but it ultimately contributes greatly to the adolescent's sense of self, as well as providing a source of pleasure, bonding, and enhancement of human relationships.[1]

Approximately 10% of youth in the United States report a physical, developmental, or sensory disability.[2] The global prevalence of intellectual disability (ID), defined as IQ less than 70 to 75, is estimated at 1%, with most being in the mild range.[3] Children and

The authors have no commercial/financial relationships to disclose.
[a] Section of Adolescent Medicine, Nationwide Children's Hospital, The Ohio State University College of Medicine, 700 Children's Drive, Columbus, OH 43205, USA; [b] Obstetrics and Gynecology, University of Michigan Medical School, 1500 East Medical Center Drive, Women's L 4000, Ann Arbor, MI 48109, USA
* Corresponding author.
E-mail address: Cynthia.Holland-Hall@NationwideChildrens.org

http://dx.doi.org/10.1016/j.pcl.2016.11.011
pediatric.theclinics.com

adolescents with disabilities have the same rights as those without disabilities,[4] but many of these adolescents face challenges to the attainment of their right to healthy sexual development.

Historically, society has ignored or minimized the issue of sexuality in persons with disabilities. Beyond the deplorable eugenics movement of the early twentieth century, during which thousands of persons with disabilities underwent involuntary sterilization, practices of institutionalization and segregation persisted, limiting the opportunity for normal psychosocial development. Today, most children and adolescents with disabilities attend schools where they interact with typically developing (TD) peers during some or all of the school day, and adults are more likely to live and work in community settings. Nevertheless, when it comes to seeing disabled persons as sexual beings, society may still perceive them negatively and stereotypically, either as asexual or as hypersexual and unable to control their sexual urges.[5,6] Medical education typically offers little instruction to new physicians on how to support and foster healthy sexuality in persons with disabilities.[7] Pediatricians are ideally suited to address these needs in youth with disabilities just as they support other aspects of normal adolescent growth and development.

ADOLESCENTS WITH PHYSICAL DISABILITIES

Adolescents with physical disabilities generally express positive desires, attitudes, and expectations about future sexual relationships.[8] Although some studies suggest positive self-esteem,[9] others indicate that persons with physical disabilities, particularly more severe impairments, experience poor body image, lower emotional well-being, and lower sexual self-esteem and satisfaction.[10] In the National Longitudinal Study of Adolescent Health (Add Health), male and female high school students with mild physical disabilities reported higher rates of same-sex attraction than their unaffected peers.[11] Attitudes toward sex were similar for girls with and without physical disabilities; however, those with disabilities reported more positive views toward pregnancy.

Socially, adolescents with physical disabilities report that they engage in less dating and fewer social activities than unaffected adolescents.[9] Nonetheless, most studies find no significant differences in self-reported history of sexual intercourse or age of first sexual intercourse in physically disabled adolescents compared with their peers.[11–13] In the Add Health study, adolescents with physical disabilities reported rates of sexual activity that were actually somewhat higher than their peers; unfortunately, for girls this reflected higher rates of both consensual and forced sex.[11] Several other studies have similarly described increased reporting of dating violence and sexual abuse and assault in physically disabled persons.[8,13,14] Adolescents with physical disabilities express concerns and a desire to discuss their sexuality with health professionals, but are less likely to have those conversations than their unaffected peers.[8,15]

Cerebral Palsy

In a review focusing on social and sexual relationships of adolescents and young adults with cerebral palsy and normal intelligence, Wiegerink and colleagues[16] found that romantic and sexual relationships were considered important but challenging to develop. These youth reported fewer social relationships, and delayed onset and lower frequency of dating. They report less experience with intimate relationships and sexual activity than their unaffected peers.[17] Adults with cerebral palsy express a desire for more education on sexuality.[18]

Myelomeningocele

Most adolescents with myelomeningocele indicate a desire to engage in sexual relationships, marry, and have children.[19,20] Cromer and colleagues[19] found that 28% of adolescents with myelomeningocele had engaged in sexual activity, compared with 60% of healthy controls. A more recent study of affected adolescents and young adults 16 to 25 years old found that 70% desired sexual contact, and 47% reported sexual contact,[21] again reflecting significantly less sexual activity than their age-matched peers without disability. Young people with myelomeningocele express a strong desire for more information on sexual function.[20] They report exposure to basic sex education, but receive very little that is specific to their condition.[21] They express concerns about urinary incontinence and may wish to explore ways to achieve sexual pleasure if genital sensation is diminished, yet they are unlikely to initiate conversations about these concerns.[19,21] Adolescent girls with myelomeningocele are usually fertile, but report low rates of contraception use and preconception counseling.[19,22] This finding is particularly concerning, given the increased risk to a woman with myelomeningocele of bearing a child with a neural tube defect.

ADOLESCENTS WITH INTELLECTUAL AND DEVELOPMENTAL DISABILITIES

Many adolescents and adults with ID describe their desires and aspirations for intimate relationships, sexual activity, and marriage.[23,24] There is some inconsistency seen in reports of sexual activity in persons with ID, likely due to methodological differences in case definition and data collection between studies. In the Add Health study, adolescents with low cognitive abilities reported increased same-sex attraction and fewer experiences of romantic attraction and vaginal intercourse than TD adolescents; those who were sexually experienced reported lower rates of contraception use and higher rates of pregnancy and sexually transmitted infection (STI).[25] In a clinical sample of adolescents with ID, Chamberlain and colleagues[26] found that adolescent girls with mild-moderate ID reported rates of sexual activity comparable to that in the TD adolescent population; they, too, demonstrated increased rates of pregnancy. In a nationally representative survey of youth in the United States, Shandra and colleagues[12] found that boys with learning disabilities or emotional disabilities were more likely to report having sex at younger ages and less likely to use condoms than other boys. Although precise estimates may be lacking, it is clear that sexual activity and its consequences are prevalent among adolescents with ID, particularly among those with mild-moderate disability.

Autism Spectrum Disorders

The social skills deficits and other features characteristic of autism spectrum disorders (ASD) may have a profound effect on sexual development; this challenge is further exacerbated in persons with cooccurrence of ID. Studies of high-functioning persons with ASD suggest differences in the experience of gender compared with control populations. Both adolescent boys and girls with ASD are more likely to be gender nonconforming and less likely to identify as heterosexual than TD peers.[27,28] Adolescent boys with high-functioning ASD report lifetime sexual experiences comparable to their TD peers, with one-third reporting having had sex with a female partner.[29,30] However, they report a lower frequency of experience with noncoital partnered sexual activity (eg, kissing, petting).[30] Parents tended to underestimate their sons' sexual experiences.[31] Adults with ASD report a later age of sexual debut and lower rates of sexual experience, interest, and arousal than the typical adult population.[27,28]

Not surprisingly, persons with ASD report challenges in the social aspects of sexual development and expression. They describe challenges with the process and expectations of courtship, and sending or receiving messages indicating interest in another.[27] Boys with ASD are more likely than their TD peers to express regret after their first sexual experience.[30] Adults describe challenges of sensory dysregulation during sexual contact, which may negatively impact the experience for both partners.[27] A subset of persons with ASD demonstrates higher rates of problematic sexual behaviors, including inappropriate romantic gestures toward others, public displays of arousal, masturbation, or exhibitionism (see later discussion).[32]

Inappropriate Sexual Behaviors

The cognitive and psychosocial skills of a youth with ID may lag significantly behind their physical maturity and sexual impulses. This discordance may lead to inappropriate sexual behaviors and subsequent societal discomfort. Public nudity, public masturbation, inappropriate handling of used menstrual products, and a general failure to recognize and respect personal boundaries may contribute to the stigma and exclusion from social activities often experienced by persons with ID. Adolescents with ID may spend play time with younger children, because they may share an interest in the same activities; inappropriate sexual behavior in this setting can lead to exclusion at best, and possibly involvement of child protection authorities.

Masturbation may be an appropriate outlet for sexual feelings and urges, and adolescents who engage in this should not be shamed or reprimanded when it occurs in the appropriate context and private setting. Interventions may be appropriate when masturbation is performed in public or is a frequent response to boredom or lack of stimulation, or if it takes the place of other, more prosocial activities. Behavioral management and sexuality education are the first-line treatments for inappropriate sexual or hypersexual behaviors. Pharmacologic intervention has been described, but is not recommended for routine use.[33]

Sexual Abuse and Exploitation

It is well documented that youth with ID are at elevated risk of sexual abuse.[11,26,34] Their desire for acceptance and conformity with TD peers may make them vulnerable to sexual exploitation, and they may have difficulty distinguishing between appropriate and inappropriate physical contact. They may lack the knowledge and communication skills needed to report abuse, or fear the consequences of disclosure.[35] Adolescent boys with ID who were formerly abused themselves are at increased risk of perpetrating inappropriate sexual acts.[34]

Caregivers' Perspectives and Influence

It is understandable that caregivers of persons with ID express significant caution and concern when confronted with issues of sexuality. Parents tend to underestimate their ID child's sexual activity and interest in sexual relationships.[23,36] Mothers of young people with ID may acknowledge the importance of addressing their child's sexuality,[37,38] yet remain hesitant to initiate conversations about sex, intimate relationships, and contraception relative to mothers of TD youth. They express fear that discussing sex may encourage inappropriate sexual behavior, and that their child may not have the coping skills to deal with sexuality.[36,37] The dissonance between perceived importance and parental behavior may be addressed through improved parental education and support.[39]

Far from being protective, the hesitation of parents and caregivers to address a child's sexuality may have a significant negative impact on psychosexual development.

Caregivers' silence on the issue suggests that sexuality is taboo; this may make the adolescent hesitant to seek information or ask questions about sex when they arise. Conversations that focus only on the negative aspects of sex may lead to negative views of sexuality that are internalized, contributing to a negative sexual self-concept and lower self-esteem.[10] Adults with ID are more likely to report negative perceptions of sex and touch as wrong and unsafe.[40] Women with ID are particularly likely to express these negative views, including fear of the sexual act, perceived lack of sexual pleasure, and fear of negative consequences of sex.[24,41] An adolescent who is deprived of appropriate information and support of healthy sexuality may be more likely to engage in inappropriate sexual behaviors.

SEXUALITY EDUCATION

Numerous studies have demonstrated the lack of adequate sexuality education provided to adolescents and adults with ID.[7,40,42,43] The traditional "Sex Ed" curriculum provided to adolescents in the United States is heterogeneous at best: the quality and quantity of information provided are variable; information may be narrowly focused on sexual behaviors and their negative consequences; content is often based on a heteronormative framework and promotes gender stereotypes. The unique needs of the adolescent with a physical or intellectual disability are unlikely to be met.

Many formal curricula for persons with ID have been developed, and some have demonstrated an increase in knowledge among participants.[39] However, none have been rigorously tested and validated with regard to their effect on sexual behavior and decision making.[39,44] Outstanding resources for both formal and informal education on sexuality for persons with disabilities are available online.[45,46] Components of an appropriate curriculum are listed in **Box 1.**

Perhaps the even bigger challenge, however, is the inherent limitation of any formal curriculum to truly inform one's understanding of sexuality. Much of what typical adolescents learn about sexuality is ultimately experiential, occurring in natural learning environments rather than a classroom. Young people grow up surrounded by both

---

Box 1
Components of a sexuality education program for youth with disabilities

- Content
  - Simple but accurate terms for anatomy
  - Physical boundaries
  - Negotiating sexual situations
  - Understanding and avoidance of sexual abuse and exploitation
  - Same-sex and opposite-sex attraction
  - Healthy sexual interactions (intercourse and noncoital alternatives)
  - Assertiveness training (saying "No")
  - Safer sexual practices
  - Pregnancy prevention

- Educational approach
  - Strength-based versus deficit-based approach
  - Simple, explicit, concrete language
  - Use of pictures, anatomically correct dolls
  - Frequent repetition
  - Adaptability for developmental levels and health literacy
  - Practice and role playing
  - Incorporate experiential learning
  - Avoidance of heteronormative approach

positive and negative sexual messages and media images that they internalize and process on conscious and subconscious levels. They engage with peers and romantic partners in both supervised and unsupervised settings, experimenting, gaining experience, and learning from their successes and mistakes. These experiences, along with formal education, religious and family values, and numerous other factors, are ultimately incorporated into the adolescent's sexual self-concept.

Adolescents with ID may lack the cognitive skills to process the abstract and often conflicting messages in their environment. In those with medical comorbidities, experiences with examinations and treatment may impact their perceptions regarding privacy and physical boundaries. They infrequently see persons with disabilities portrayed in the media as desirable romantic partners. They generally have smaller social circles than TD adolescents.[43] Caregivers, through appropriate and well-intentioned efforts to limit the risk of harm, may place strict limitations on social interactions and activities, particularly those with reduced levels of supervision. The disabled adolescent's opportunities for experiential learning are limited, and those experiences are often disproportionately negative. In contrast to supporting healthy sexual development, caregivers may inadvertently impair psychosocial and sexual development by restricting opportunities for sexual exploration. This limitation of experiential learning may ultimately lead to a worse sexual self-concept and poor sexual decision-making skills in adulthood.

THE ROLE OF THE MEDICAL PROVIDER
Puberty and Menstruation

Puberty typically occurs within the expected timeframe, particularly for adolescents with an isolated congenital or acquired physical disability or idiopathic ID. Children with certain genetic syndromes or neurodevelopmental disabilities, including neural tube defects or major brain malformations, may experience premature adrenarche or pubarche. In many, these remain isolated changes; in others, they may progress to true precocious puberty.[47,48] For children who have experienced nutritional deficiencies or failure to reach expected growth parameters due to their condition, puberty may occur later.[47] Girls with ASD also may undergo somewhat delayed puberty and menarche.[49]

Menstruation can be challenging for girls with special needs. They may need assistance changing pads, due to dexterity issues caused by physical disabilities, or limited understanding of the process in girls with ID. Pain and irregular bleeding, common in teenagers, may cause a significant burden for the patient and her caregivers, or limit her ability to participate in school or other activities. Most families learn to manage menstruation effectively, even for teens with severe disability.[50,51] The medical provider should initiate anticipatory guidance about the menstrual periods once breast development starts, because there is typically 2 to 3 years between thelarche and the onset of menses. Hormonal treatment to prevent menarche, sometimes requested by caregivers, is generally not recommended because this may limit ongoing normal growth. Allowing menarche to occur also gives families an opportunity to see how the experience of the menstrual cycle affects the adolescent. Tips for managing menstrual periods are presented in **Box 2**.

When hormonal contraception is considered, the desired outcomes should be clarified, because this may affect the method choice. For example, the goal may be to prevent pregnancy, to decrease heavy bleeding, to eliminate menstrual cramps, or to attempt to obtain amenorrhea. Families must understand that complete amenorrhea is almost impossible, so period and pad education remains critical.[52,53]

Box 2
Tips for managing menstruation in girls with intellectual disabilities

- Avoid negative references to menstruation; discuss menstruation as a normal part of growing up.
- Discuss and practice pad use *prior to* menstruation.
- Use an alarm or reminder system to signal time for a pad change.
- Create a checklist for steps involved in changing pads (eg, remove, wrap up, and discard used pad; wash hands, and so forth).
- Consider the use of a sticker chart or reward system for good hygiene practices.
- For patients using a diaper, a pad placed within the diaper may facilitate easier changes and save money.
- Consider allowing patient to observe a relative or close female friend managing menstrual hygiene, if comfortable.
- Track periods on a calendar to anticipate next menses.

Medical Interventions

1. *Nonsteroidal anti-inflammatory drugs* can be used to treat menstrual cramps and may decrease the menstrual flow when taken consistently.[54] Gastrointestinal and neurologic side effects may limit their use.[55]
2. The *combination estrogen-progesterone containing methods* are used extensively in adolescents with disabilities[56] and can be used either cyclically or in an extended or continuous fashion to decrease the frequency of menstrual cycles.[57]
   a. *Combined Oral Contraceptives (COC)*. Daily oral use is paramount because intermittent use is associated with breakthrough bleeding. For teens with swallowing issues, one chewable product is currently available. Extended use (with elimination of the "placebo" pills) has been described, providing good cycle control[58]; however, unpredictable bleeding remains a side effect, whether a fixed or a flexible extended regimen is used.[59]
   b. *Transdermal combined hormones*. The weekly contraceptive patch can be used either cyclically or with extended use; extended use provides similar or better cycle control than COC.[60] For patients with ID who may remove the patch inappropriately, the patch may be placed on difficult-to-reach places, such as the upper back.
   c. *Vaginal ring*. The monthly vaginal ring can be used cyclically or extended in an off-label use. It provides equivalent cycle control to COC.[61] This method, however, has limited utility for teens with disabilities, because the ring needs to be placed intravaginally, which requires a fair amount of manual dexterity and coordination. If the adolescent cannot do this herself, there are clear privacy concerns.
3. *Progesterone-only methods*
   a. The *progesterone-only contraceptive pill (POP)* has a significant side effect of irregular bleeding, because the short half-life of norethindrone makes exact 24-hour compliance imperative. Amenorrhea is achieved in about only 10% of women. Therefore, its use is limited for menstrual management. Higher doses of norethindrone, medroxyprogesterone, and megestrol have been used to treat heavy menstrual cycles in older women with some positive results, and may be considered if amenorrhea is desired.[52]

b. *Depot medroxyprogesterone acetate*, the 12-week intramuscular or subcutaneous injection, is a good form of menstrual management with a high rate of amenorrhea (around 50% at 12 months).[62] However, 2 potential side effects have contributed to declining use in the disabled population.[56] DMPA may contribute to weight gain. A review of the available studies showed overall weight gain is not excessive; however, the risk is greatest in overweight teenagers. Because this weight gain often is apparent after the first 3 months, discontinuation for teens with significant weight gain at that time should be considered.[63] Weight gain significantly affects the health and the ability of a teen to do her own wheelchair transfers or for caregivers to lift her. DMPA also may interfere with the normal bone density gain in early adolescence.[64] Many patients with disabilities already have compromised bone density due to poor nutrition, use of anticonvulsants, reduced mobility, and possible vitamin D deficiency.[47] Studies suggest that the bone loss can be regained after stopping DMPA; however, many teens with ID stay on it for a prolonged period of time. Adequate calcium and vitamin D may be helpful.[65]

c. *Subdermal implant.* The 3-year single-rod etonogestrel implant provides excellent contraception; however, because of an unfavorable irregular bleeding pattern and amenorrhea rates of only 20% at 1 year, the implant is usually not recommended for menstrual management. Insertion and removal require patient cooperation, which may be challenging for some teenagers with ID. However, for those teens who can deal with the intermittent bleeding and desire excellent birth control, this remains a viable option.[66]

d. The *Levonorgestrel intrauterine device (LNG-IUD)* provides excellent contraceptive efficacy as well as good cycle control for bleeding and cramping. In the general adolescent population, it has recently become more popular, endorsed as a first-line method by the American College of Obstetricians and Gynecologists (ACOG).[67,68] In teens with disabilities, the LNG-IUD has been described in several studies with normal expulsion rates, normal removal rates for pain and bleeding, and a 70% amenorrhea rate in girls for whom that information was noted.[56,69–71] General anesthesia is often used for placement. Preinsertion ultrasonography is not routinely indicated.[72] The copper IUD, associated with increased bleeding and cramping, is not useful for menstrual management.

All estrogen-containing medications increase the risk of venous thromboembolism (VTE), from 2.1/10,000 to 4/10,000 in adolescent COC users. The risk for patch and ring users may be slightly higher.[73] Risk is increased with higher dose of estrogen, obesity, smoking, and a familial clotting disorder. Whether different progestins have different rates of VTE remains controversial. Registry studies suggest a slightly lower risk of VTE for first- and second-generation progestins, but this was not found in cohort studies.[74] Whether the use of a wheelchair increases the VTE risk is unknown, but it has not been reported in adolescents. It is prudent to discuss these concerns with the patient and her family and assess for additional risk factors, and if the decision is to use an estrogen containing method, to use a lower dose estrogen with a first- or second-generation progestin. The risk of VTE in progesterone-only methods appears to be very low.[75]

Surgical Interventions

Endometrial ablation is a procedure designed to destroy the endometrial lining in women who have completed childbearing. In about 25% to 40% of women, this results in amenorrhea. In women less than the age of 35, 31% required another procedure within 5 years, compared with less than 10% over than the age of 45. Because ablation renders women less fertile, it can be considered a sterilization procedure with possible legal implications. Both the ACOG and the American Academy of Pediatrics (AAP) have stated that ablation is not recommended in teens.[76,77] Caregivers may inquire about hysterectomy to achieve amenorrhea and pregnancy prevention. Concerns include both surgical complications and ethical and legal implications for those patients who cannot give their own consent. A hysterectomy for no other indication than eliminating menstrual periods and the chance of pregnancy has not been endorsed by ACOG and AAP.[76,77]

Supporting Healthy Sexuality

By addressing the same aspects of sexual development and sexual health care needs present in TD youth (**Box 3**), the provider emphasizes the normative aspects of sexual development in disabled youth. The provider may point out that many ID young adults ultimately have the capacity to engage in sexual activity of some sort. The planning, experiences, and educational efforts made during adolescence may provide the adult with more tools to make healthy decisions. Although protecting the child from harm remains of utmost importance, this must be balanced, to the extent possible, with facilitating developmentally appropriate discussions and experiences that permit learning and foster healthy sexual development. Anticipatory guidance for persons with disabilities (**Box 4**) includes many of the same approaches recommended for TD children, such as starting conversations about sexuality early, repeating them often, and using "teachable moments" as they arise in real life and in the media.

The clinician should model involving patients in their own health care to the extent that they are developmentally capable. Genital examinations should be performed

---

Box 3
Supporting healthy sexual development in adolescents with developmental disabilities: the role of the medical provider

- Emphasize sexual development as a normative experience
  - Discuss both positive and negative aspects
  - Approach as you would with all patients at a similar developmental level

- Include external genital examinations in routine physicals
  - Demonstrate respect for privacy and dignity
  - Use as "teachable moment" for appropriate and inappropriate touch
  - Set stage for reproductive care in adulthood

- Discuss behavioral and hormonal approaches to managing menstruation

- For sexually active patients
  - Provide or refer for contraception
  - Perform STI testing using urine or vaginal swab
  - Refer for genetic counseling if indicated
  - Folic acid supplementation for adolescent girl (4 mg daily for adolescents with myelomeningocele; 0.4–1 mg daily for others)

- Screen for sexual abuse and consider in patients presenting with behavior changes or genitourinary/bowel symptoms

- Vaccinate against HPV

- Screen for depression, anxiety, and substance use

- Provide anticipatory guidance on healthy sexual development throughout childhood and adolescence (see **Box 4**)

Box 4
Supporting healthy sexual development in adolescents with developmental disabilities: anticipatory guidance for caregivers

- Begin in early childhood
  - Role model appropriate degrees of modesty, privacy
  - "Public" versus "private" behaviors
  - Role model healthy sexual expression

- Start conversations early and repeat often
  - Approach sequentially (eg, body parts → boundaries → puberty → sexual behaviors) at the pace that is right for your child
  - Speak frankly and concretely
  - Ask about questions or concerns

- Respond calmly to questions about sex
  - Do not demonstrate anger or shock
  - Use as an opportunity to explore the adolescent's thoughts and experiences
  - "What makes you ask that question?"
  - "Where did you learn that word?"

- Use teachable moments (real life and media) to facilitate discussion and reinforce appropriate behavior

- Prepare female children for menstruation
  - Discuss ahead of time
  - Distinguish menstrual blood from bleeding caused by injury
  - Model menstrual hygiene if comfortable doing so
  - Consider use of reminders, sticker charts, rewards to support menstrual hygiene practices

- Acknowledge that many with intellectual disability ultimately have the desire and decisional capacity to choose to engage in sexual activity

- Provide opportunities for healthy sexual development while limiting risk of harm
  - Promote normal teen activities and interactions
  - Respect need for privacy
  - Teach appropriate setting and context for masturbation
  - Provide experiential learning opportunities

- Monitor use of social media and place limits as needed

- Include sex education and social skills training in Individualized Education Program

---

routinely, using the opportunity to discuss body parts, answer questions, and pave the way for more extensive genital examinations that may be needed in adulthood. While exploring and discussing the adolescent's romantic interests and intents, the provider may remind the patient and caregivers that there are many means of sexual contact and expression that may be gratifying while presenting less risk than intercourse. A patient with a physical disability may be encouraged to consider a more diverse repertoire of opportunities for sexual expression as well.

Sexually active adolescents should be tested for Chlamydia and gonorrhea at least yearly. STI testing, using urine or a vaginal swab with a nucleic acid amplification test, is minimally invasive and has high sensitivity and specificity. Cervical cancer screening by Pap smear is recommended starting at the age of 21 years. If a young woman with disabilities cannot tolerate a pelvic examination, an assessment of her risk for cervical cancer (ie, sexual contact) is made to determine whether a pelvic examination under sedation is indicated. The possibility of human papillomavirus (HPV) screening using vaginal swabs may become applicable for this population in the future; however, current recommendations remain preliminary.[78]

SUMMARY

Sexuality is a part of human development, no less for disabled persons than for persons without disability. Some persons with disability face challenges to healthy sexual development, but with supportive medical providers and caregivers, opportunities for formal and experiential learning, and a broadened view of healthy sexual behavior and expression, these challenges can be overcome.

REFERENCES

1. Murphy NA, Elias ER. Sexuality of children and adolescents with developmental disabilities. Pediatrics 2006;118(1):398–403.
2. Brault MW. Current population reports. Washington, DC: US Census Bureau 2012;70–131.
3. Maulik PK, Mascarenhas MN, Mathers CD, et al. Prevalence of intellectual disability: a meta-analysis of population-based studies. Res Dev Disabil 2011; 32(2):419–36.
4. Council on Community Pediatrics and Committee on Native American Child Health. Policy statement-health equity and children's rights. Pediatrics 2010; 125(4):838–49.
5. Esmail S, Darry K, Walter A, et al. Attitudes and perceptions towards disability and sexuality. Disabil Rehabil 2010;32(14):1148–55.
6. Neufeld JA, Klingbeil F, Bryen DN, et al. Adolescent sexuality and disability. Phys Med Rehabil Clin N Am 2002;13(4):857–73.
7. Greenwood NW, Wilkinson J. Sexual and reproductive health care for women with intellectual disabilities: a primary care perspective. Int J Family Med 2013;2013: 642472.
8. Jemta L, Fugl-Meyer KS, Oberg K. On intimacy, sexual activities and exposure to sexual abuse among children and adolescents with mobility impairment. Acta Paediatr 2008;97(5):641–6.
9. Stevens SE, Steele CA, Jutai JW, et al. Adolescents with physical disabilities: some psychosocial aspects of health. J Adolesc Health 1996;19(2):157–64.
10. McCabe MP, Taleporos G. Sexual esteem, sexual satisfaction, and sexual behavior among people with physical disability. Arch Sex Behav 2003;32(4): 359–69.
11. Cheng MM, Udry JR. Sexual behaviors of physically disabled adolescents in the United States. J Adolesc Health 2002;31(1):48–58.
12. Shandra CL, Shameem M, Ghori SJ. Disability and the context of boys' first sexual intercourse. J Adolesc Health 2016;58(3):302–9.
13. Suris JC, Resnick MD, Cassuto N, et al. Sexual behavior of adolescents with chronic disease and disability. J Adolesc Health 1996;19(2):124–31.
14. Mitra M, Mouradian VE, McKenna M. Dating violence and associated health risks among high school students with disabilities. Matern Child Health J 2013;17(6): 1088–94.
15. Seburg EM, McMorris BJ, Garwick AW, et al. Disability and discussions of health-related behaviors between youth and health care providers. J Adolesc Health 2015;57(1):81–6.
16. Wiegerink DJ, Roebroeck ME, Donkervoort M, et al. Social and sexual relationships of adolescents and young adults with cerebral palsy: a review. Clin Rehabil 2006;20(12):1023–31.

17. Wiegerink DJ, Roebroeck ME, Donkervoort M, et al. Social, intimate and sexual relationships of adolescents with cerebral palsy compared with able-bodied age-mates. J Rehabil Med 2008;40(2):112–8.

18. Cho SR, Park ES, Park CI, et al. Characteristics of psychosexual functioning in adults with cerebral palsy. Clin Rehabil 2004;18(4):423–9.

19. Cromer BA, Enrile B, McCoy K, et al. Knowledge, attitudes and behavior related to sexuality in adolescents with chronic disability. Dev Med Child Neurol 1990; 32(7):602–10.

20. Lindehall B, Moller A, Hjalmas K, et al. Psychosocial factors in teenagers and young adults with myelomeningocele and clean intermittent catheterization. Scand J Urol Nephrol 2008;42(6):539–44.

21. Verhoef M, Barf HA, Vroege JA, et al. Sex education, relationships, and sexuality in young adults with spina bifida. Arch Phys Med Rehabil 2005;86(5):979–87.

22. Visconti D, Noia G, Triarico S, et al. Sexuality, pre-conception counseling and urological management of pregnancy for young women with spina bifida. Eur J Obstet Gynecol Reprod Biol 2012;163(2):129–33.

23. Healy E, McGuire BE, Evans DS, et al. Sexuality and personal relationships for people with an intellectual disability. Part I: service-user perspectives. J Intellect Disabil Res 2009;53(11):905–12.

24. Siebelink EM, de Jong MD, Taal E, et al. Sexuality and people with intellectual disabilities: assessment of knowledge, attitudes, experiences, and needs. Ment Retard 2006;44(4):283–94.

25. Cheng MM, Udry JR. Sexual experiences of adolescents with low cognitive abilities in the US. J Dev Phys Disabil 2005;17(2):155–72.

26. Chamberlain A, Rauh J, Passer A, et al. Issues in fertility control for mentally retarded female adolescents: I. Sexual activity, sexual abuse, and contraception. Pediatrics 1984;73(4):445–50.

27. Barnett JP, Maticka-Tyndale E. Qualitative exploration of sexual experiences among adults on the autism spectrum: implications for sex education. Perspect Sex Reprod Health 2015;47(4):171–9.

28. Bejerot S, Eriksson JM. Sexuality and gender role in autism spectrum disorder: a case control study. PLoS One 2014;9(1):e87961.

29. Dewinter J, Vermeiren R, Vanwesenbeeck I, et al. Sexuality in adolescent boys with autism spectrum disorder: self-reported behaviours and attitudes. J Autism Dev Disord 2015;45(3):731–41.

30. Dewinter J, Vermeiren R, Vanwesenbeeck I, et al. Adolescent boys with autism spectrum disorder growing up: follow-up of self-reported sexual experience. Eur Child Adolesc Psychiatry 2016;25(9):969–78.

31. Dewinter J, Vermeiren R, Vanwesenbeeck I, et al. Parental awareness of sexual experience in adolescent boys with autism spectrum disorder. J Autism Dev Disord 2016;46(2):713–9.

32. Beddows N, Brooks R. Inappropriate sexual behaviour in adolescents with autism spectrum disorder: what education is recommended and why. Early Interv Psychiatry 2016;10(4):282–9.

33. Sajith SG, Morgan C, Clarke D. Pharmacological management of inappropriate sexual behaviours: a review of its evidence, rationale and scope in relation to men with intellectual disabilities. J Intellect Disabil Res 2008;52(12):1078–90.

34. Wissink IB, van Vugt E, Moonen X, et al. Sexual abuse involving children with an intellectual disability (ID): a narrative review. Res Dev Disabil 2015;36:20–35.

35. Miller HL, Pavlik KM, Kim MA, et al. An exploratory study of the knowledge of personal safety skills among children with developmental disabilities and their parents. J Appl Res Intellect Disabil 2016. [Epub ahead of print].

36. Cheng MM, Udry JR. How much do mentally disabled adolescents know about sex and birth control. Adolesc Fam Health 2003;3(1):28–38.

37. Pownall JD, Jahoda A, Hastings R, et al. Sexual understanding and development of young people with intellectual disabilities: mothers' perspectives of within-family context. Am J Intellect Dev Disabil 2011;116(3):205–19.

38. Swango-Wilson A. Caregiver perceptions and implications for sex education for individuals with intellectual and developmental disabilities. Sex Disabil 2008; 26(3):167–74.

39. McGuire BE, Bayley AA. Relationships, sexuality and decision-making capacity in people with an intellectual disability. Curr Opin Psychiatry 2011;24(5):398–402.

40. McCabe MP. Sexual knowledge, experience and feelings among people with disability. Sex Disabil 1999;17(2):157–70.

41. Bernert DJ, Ogletree RJ. Women with intellectual disabilities talk about their perceptions of sex. J Intellect Disabil Res 2013;57(3):240–9.

42. Barnard-Brak L, Schmidt M, Chesnut S, et al. Predictors of access to sex education for children with intellectual disabilities in public schools. Intellect Dev Disabil 2014;52(2):85–97.

43. Jahoda A, Pownall J. Sexual understanding, sources of information and social networks; the reports of young people with intellectual disabilities and their non-disabled peers. J Intellect Disabil Res 2014;58(5):430–41.

44. Doughty AH, Kane LM. Teaching abuse-protection skills to people with intellectual, disabilities: a review of the literature. Res Dev Disabil 2010;31(2):331–7.

45. Available at: http://www.mass.gov/eohhs/docs/dph/com-health/prevention/hrhs-sexuality-and-disability-resource-guide.pdf. Accessed December 7, 2016.

46. Available at: http://disability-abuse.com/. Accessed December 7, 2016.

47. Zacharin M. Endocrine problems in children and adolescents who have disabilities. Horm Res Paediatr 2013;80(4):221–8.

48. Siddiqi SU, Van Dyke DC, Donohoue P, et al. Premature sexual development in individuals with neurodevelopmental disabilities. Dev Med Child Neurol 1999; 41(6):392–5.

49. Knickmeyer RC, Wheelwright S, Hoekstra R, et al. Age of menarche in females with autism spectrum conditions. Dev Med Child Neurol 2006;48(12):1007–8.

50. Kaskowitz AP, Dendrinos M, Murray PJ, et al. The effect of menstrual issues on young women with Angelman syndrome. J Pediatr Adolesc Gynecol 2016; 29(4):348–52.

51. Hamilton A, Marshal MP, Sucato GS, et al. Rett syndrome and menstruation. J Pediatr Adolesc Gynecol 2012;25(2):122–6.

52. Altshuler AL, Hillard PJ. Menstrual suppression for adolescents. Curr Opin Obstet Gynecol 2014;26(5):323–31.

53. Abdel-Aleem H, d'Arcangues C, Vogelsong KM, et al. Treatment of vaginal bleeding irregularities induced by progestin only contraceptives. Cochrane Database Syst Rev 2013;(10):CD003449.

54. Lethaby A, Duckitt K, Farquhar C. Non-steroidal anti-inflammatory drugs for heavy menstrual bleeding. Cochrane Database Syst Rev 2013;(1):CD000400.

55. Marjoribanks J, Ayeleke RO, Farquhar C, et al. Nonsteroidal anti-inflammatory drugs for dysmenorrhoea. Cochrane Database Syst Rev 2015;(7):CD001751.

56. Kirkham YA, Allen L, Kives S, et al. Trends in menstrual concerns and suppression in adolescents with developmental disabilities. J Adolesc Health 2013; 53(3):407–12.

57. Jacobson JC, Likis FE, Murphy PA. Extended and continuous combined contraceptive regimens for menstrual suppression. J Midwifery Womens Health 2012; 57(6):585–92.

58. Edelman A, Micks E, Gallo MF, et al. Continuous or extended cycle vs. cyclic use of combined hormonal contraceptives for contraception. Cochrane Database Syst Rev 2014;(7):CD004695.

59. Han L, Jensen JT. Expert opinion on a flexible extended regimen of drospirenone/ethinyl estradiol contraceptive. Expert Opin Pharmacother 2014;15(14):2071–9.

60. Stewart FH, Kaunitz AM, Laguardia KD, et al. Extended use of transdermal norelgestromin/ethinyl estradiol: a randomized trial. Obstet Gynecol 2005;105(6): 1389–96.

61. Weisberg E, Merki-Feld GS, McGeechan K, et al. Randomized comparison of bleeding patterns in women using a combined contraceptive vaginal ring or a low-dose combined oral contraceptive on a menstrually signaled regimen. Contraception 2015;91(2):121–6.

62. Hubacher D, Lopez L, Steiner MJ, et al. Menstrual pattern changes from levonorgestrel subdermal implants and DMPA: systematic review and evidence-based comparisons. Contraception 2009;80(2):113–8.

63. Lopez LM, Edelman A, Chen M, et al. Progestin-only contraceptives: effects on weight. Cochrane Database Syst Rev 2013;(7):CD008815.

64. American College of Obstetricians and Gynecologists. Committee opinion no. 602: Depot medroxyprogesterone acetate and bone effects. Obstet Gynecol 2014;123(6):1398–402.

65. Rahman M, Berenson AB. Predictors of higher bone mineral density loss and use of depot medroxyprogesterone acetate. Obstet Gynecol 2010;115(1):35–40.

66. Mansour D, Korver T, Marintcheva-Petrova M, et al. The effects of Implanon on menstrual bleeding patterns. Eur J Contracept Reprod Health Care 2008; 13(Suppl 1):13–28.

67. Committee on Adolescent Health Care Long-Acting Reversible Contraception Working Group, The American College of Obstetricians and Gynecologists. Committee opinion no. 539: adolescents and long-acting reversible contraception: implants and intrauterine devices. Obstet Gynecol 2012;120(4):983–8.

68. American Academy of Pediatrics, The Committee on Adolescence. Contraception for adolescents. Pediatrics 2014;134(4):e1244–1256.

69. Hillard PJ. Menstrual suppression with the levonorgestrel intrauterine system in girls with developmental delay. J Pediatr Adolesc Gynecol 2012;25(5):308–13.

70. Pillai M, O'Brien K, Hill E. The levonorgestrel intrauterine system (Mirena) for the treatment of menstrual problems in adolescents with medical disorders, or physical or learning disabilities. BJOG 2010;117(2):216–21.

71. Savasi I, Jayasinghe K, Moore P, et al. Complication rates associated with levonorgestrel intrauterine system use in adolescents with developmental disabilities. J Pediatr Adolesc Gynecol 2014;27(1):25–8.

72. Whyte H, Pecchioli Y, Oyewumi L, et al. Uterine length in adolescents with developmental disability: are ultrasounds necessary prior to insertion of the levonorgestrel intrauterine system? J Pediatr Adolesc Gynecol 2016;26(6):648–52.

73. Hugon-Rodin J, Gompel A, Plu-Bureau G. Epidemiology of hormonal contraceptives-related venous thromboembolism. Eur J Endocrinol 2014;171(6):R221–30.

74. Han L, Jensen JT. Does the progestogen used in combined hormonal contraception affect venous thrombosis risk? Obstet Gynecol Clin North Am 2015;42(4): 683–98.
75. Tepper NK, Whiteman MK, Marchbanks PA, et al. Progestin-only contraception and thromboembolism: a systematic review. Contraception 2016;94:678–700.
76. American College of Obstetricians and Gynecologists Committee on Adolescent Health Care. ACOG Committee opinion no. 448: menstrual manipulation for adolescents with disabilities. Obstet Gynecol 2009;114(6):1428–31.
77. Quint EH, O'Brien RF, AAP The Committee on Adolescence, et al. Menstrual management for adolescents with disabilities. Pediatrics 2016;137(4):e20160295.
78. Huh WK, Ault KA, Chelmow D, et al. Use of primary high-risk human papillomavirus testing for cervical cancer screening: interim clinical guidance. Obstet Gynecol 2015;125(2):330–7.

Treating Youths in the Juvenile Justice System

Ann L. Sattler, MD, MAT

KEYWORDS

- Juvenile justice • Detained girls • Sexual risk-taking • STIs • Juvenile detention

KEY POINTS

- Juvenile justice-involved youths reside primarily in the community and receive health care from community providers.
- Adolescents involved with the correctional system report more high-risk sexual behaviors that lead to disproportionate rates of negative health outcomes.
- Pediatric providers are uniquely positioned to identify and address high-risk sexual behaviors and comorbid substance abuse and mental health issues in this underserved population.

Approximately 70,800 US youths were housed in more than 2500 juvenile justice (JJ) residential placement facilities nationwide according to the most recent statistics from the Office of Juvenile Justice and Delinquency Prevention.[1,2] Despite 25 years of movement away from juvenile incarceration toward decriminalization and diversion to community-based programs, the United States still incarcerates a higher percentage of youths than any other developed country.[3] However, most of the 2 million juveniles arrested and processed by the courts are remanded to community programs or probation.[4] Higher rates of risky sexual and substance use behaviors reported by JJ-involved youths, compared with noninvolved peers, present the community with public health risks. High rates of recidivism mean that there is often a revolving door through which many JJ-involved youths shuttle between detention and home communities. One-fifth of youths remanded to JJ residential placements were returned to the community in less than 2 weeks, and many return to detention repeatedly.[1,5,6]

Pediatricians are in a unique position to address factors that place children at risk for entry into the JJ system and to provide continuity of care, screening, and treatment of detained youths when they return to community care. Pediatric providers are also positioned to be powerful advocates for social policy changes and funding to remediate the social determinants of health (poverty, family dysfunction, substance and child abuse, and depression), which are predictors of JJ involvement.[7]

Disclosures: The author has no financial or commercial conflict of interest to disclose.
Division of Adolescent Medicine, Department of Pediatrics, University of Massachusetts Medical School, 55 Lake Avenue North, Worcester, MA 01655, USA
E-mail address: ann.sattler@umassmemorial.org

Pediatr Clin N Am 64 (2017) 451–462
http://dx.doi.org/10.1016/j.pcl.2016.11.012
0031-3955/17/© 2016 Elsevier Inc. All rights reserved.

Higher rates of sexually transmitted infections (STIs), including chlamydia, gonorrhea, syphilis, and human immunodeficiency virus (HIV), have been reported in both juveniles and adults entering correctional facilities and also in those returning to community settings. Reported rates underestimate the problem, because the lack of available testing and treatment in many juvenile facilities leads to underreporting.[8] The risk behaviors in which adolescents engage are clearly recognized as the root cause of such health outcomes.[9] Because risky sexual behaviors themselves are correlated with early death, disability, and socioeconomic challenges, they have long been recognized as a public health priority.[10] Recent national surveys of high school youths indicate that today's adolescents are reporting less frequent sexual intercourse encounters, fewer sexual partners, less substance use before sex, and increased condom and other contraceptive use.[10] However, in the JJ population, these decreases are not being seen. It is essential to address not only the sexual risk behaviors and their consequences in this population but also the individual, family, and sociodemographic factors that contributed to those behaviors.

SEXUAL RISK PERSISTS DURING AND AFTER ANY JUSTICE SYSTEM CONTACT

A longitudinal study of 1829 youths detained between 1995 and 1998 in Chicago's Cook County Juvenile Detention Center aimed to identify HIV/STI risk behaviors at baseline and again at follow-up 3.5 to 4.5 years later.[11] More than 60% engaged in 10 or more sexual risk behaviors at baseline and approximately two-thirds persisted or increased that pattern at follow-up. Of youths who reported unprotected vaginal sex at baseline, more than 50% of boys and almost 70% of girls maintained this behavior 3 to 4 years later. Having unprotected sex while drunk or high was reported at follow-up by 75% of boys and 60% of girls. More than half the study subjects had a substance use disorder at baseline, increasing at follow-up to greater than 80% use. At the time of that study, injection drug use was uncommon at both baseline and follow-up. Given that the epidemiology of HIV has shifted toward increased heterosexual transmission, accounting for one-third of current AIDS cases, up from 4% in early HIV reporting, this population is at high risk for HIV/AIDS.[12,13] Most of these behaviors were more prevalent among youths who were arrested and returned to the community, compared with those who were incarcerated, so community health providers must be part of the solution, developing comfort in communicating with high-risk youths and in using motivational interviewing to change behaviors.

Increased STI/HIV risks follow not only detention or incarceration, but also any encounters with the justice system. Police encounters or arrests may be a proxy for other factors that predict increased STI/HIV risk. A retrospective cohort study of adults and juveniles having had any contact with the Marion County, Indiana justice system looked at STI occurrence and HIV incidence rates in the year following arrest or incarceration, compared with the county's nonoffender rates.[14,15] Offender rates were higher in general, but rates for chlamydia (2968 per 100,000) and gonorrhea (2305 per 100,000) were higher than for syphilis (278 per 100,000) and HIV (61 per 100,000). Rates were up to 2.8 times higher in women than in men and 6.9 times higher in blacks than in whites. Chlamydia and gonorrhea rates were highest among 15 to 19 year olds. Incident HIV was highest in 20 to 44 year olds, suggesting likely exposure during adolescence. Interestingly, those arrested, but not detained, had higher annual rates of testing positive for these STIs in follow-up compared with those who were incarcerated, presumably because sexual activity in jail and prison is prohibited.[14]

GIRLS: A JUVENILE JUSTICE MINORITY POPULATION WITH UNIQUE RISK PROFILES

Although girls continue to comprise a minority of detained and arrested juveniles, the number of arrested and detained girls has been substantially increasing in recent years.[16,17] In 2011, girls comprised nearly 30% of all nationwide juvenile arrests.[17] Because of the increasing use of programs to divert youths arrested for minor infractions to community settings or probation, rather than lock-up, juvenile incarceration rates overall have been decreasing over the past 2 decades. However, the rate of decrease for girls (8%) has been much lower than for boys (18%), meaning that arrested girls are still disproportionately remanded to incarceration versus community diversion compared with boys.[18]

Child Abuse, Substance Use, and Mental Heath Issues Increase Girls' Sexual Risks

Girls in the JJ system are significantly more likely than boys in the system to have been victims of sexual and/or physical abuse before incarceration.[19–21] Rates of abuse in JJ-involved girls are 3.5 to 10 times higher than rates for their male counterparts.[22] These findings of significantly different male and female histories reported by youths in JJ settings suggest the need for both gender-specific and gender-sensitive female programming and PTSD/child abuse/trauma training for staff and medical providers.

Leve and colleagues[23] (2015) followed 166 JJ-involved girls from adolescence to young adulthood, reporting that a history of sexual abuse correlated with increased rates of unsafe sexual behaviors in young adulthood, which in turn was associated with acquiring an STI, putting these girls at greater risk for acquiring HIV/AIDS. Discomfort talking with partners about safer sex practices moderated the association between sexual abuse history and unsafe sex in young adulthood. Girls with a history of sexual abuse, who also have difficulty talking to partners about sex practices, reported an 8.5 times higher rate of unsafe sex practices compared with their JJ peers without sexual abuse histories.[23] Few studies have evaluated how the relationship between child abuse and sexual risk-taking functions. Lopez and colleagues[24] investigated possible mediators in the pathway leading from child maltreatment to noncondom use, a behavior usually highly correlated with other sexual risk-taking behaviors. Basing their hypotheses on the theory that females' sense of self-worth, empowerment, and identity is rooted in relationships with others, they predicted that intimate partner relationships would have a powerful impact on condom use. Although depressive self-concept and condom use self-efficacy were significantly related to noncondom use for white girls only, they were not mediators. There was evidence, for African-American girls only, that child maltreatment results in a pathway from depressive feelings and lower self-worth to substance use (self-medication), which may then lead to noncondom use.[24]

A history of sexual abuse has long been correlated with more serious delinquency compared with counterparts without that history.[25,26] It was commonly thought that childhood abuse predicted higher rates of promiscuity, teenage pregnancy, and prostitution. However, Widom and Kuhns'[27] 1996 prospective study of 1575 children referred for physical or sexual abuse between 1967 and 1971 found only the likelihood of engaging in prostitution differentiated the abused group from the nonabused group, and that finding applied only to girls. The highest rates of prostitution correlated with a history of physical abuse (12.8%), followed by sexual abuse (10.5%) and neglect (9%). Childhood sexual abuse was not found to be predictive of teenage pregnancy or promiscuity in this study.[27] Exposure to interparental violence or child abuse does increase 7-fold the likelihood that girls will commit a violent act and will be referred to JJ, compared with an age-matched community sample not exposed to domestic violence.[28] A case-controlled study of children aged 0 to 11 years, processed for child physical or sexual abuse between 1967 and 1971, followed up in 2013, reported that boys, but not girls, with histories of physical abuse were significantly at greater risk than controls for being arrested for sexual offenses (odds ratio [OR] 2.21; confidence interval, 1.38–3.40). A history of sexual abuse did not significantly predict arrest for sexual offenses (OR 2.13).[27]

Significantly higher rates of comorbid mental health problems in girls entering the JJ system add to the likelihood of risky sexual behaviors compared with non JJ-involved community peers and also compared with boys in the system.[23,29] Risky sexual behavior (multiple partners, partners injecting drugs, failure to use condoms during intercourse), prevalent among JJ-involved girls, is also associated with substance use.[23]

Higher Female Rates of Sexually Transmitted Infections and Risky Sexual Behaviors and Partners

Seventy-six percent of girls in a short-term JJ facility reported being sexually active with initial sexual experience before 14 years of age.[30] Girls in one study reported 3 or more sexual partners with 10% reporting trading sex for money during their teenage years.[31] In comparison, only 48% of high school girls in a population-based survey reported having had sexual experience and only 13% reported having 4 or more lifetime sexual partners.[32,33] An earlier study of detained girls reported that the average number of lifetime sex partners was 8.8.[34] Rates of STIs (20%–42%) discovered during health evaluations in JJ facilities, are much higher than those in community samples.[31,34]

Compared with JJ-involved boys, JJ girls are reported to have higher rates of STDs.[35–37] They are also more likely to engage in other risky sexual practices, including unprotected sex, sex with high-risk partners, and trading sex for money.[38] Compared with boys, girls in a study of teens (N = 523) in a southern US city juvenile detention center reported significantly greater knowledge, less peer influence, more positive attitudes toward condoms, higher recognition of risk of STIs, and greater self-efficacy on paper; but surprisingly they reported less actual condom use compared with male peers.[39] This gendered paradox (higher self-efficacy, yet lower condom use) may reflect negative partner attitudes toward condoms in relationships in which the boy has more power or other factors that differentially impact girls' difficulty communicating and asserting their preferences.

Girls in the JJ system tend to have older sexual partners than either male counterparts in the system or non–JJ-involved girls. One study reported that one-third of girls in a JJ facility indicated sexual involvement with a partner more than 5 years older.[30] Age difference alone usually creates a power differential; but in addition, some of these older partners may be acting as pimps, who exercise complete financial, emotional, and physical control over the girls (**Boxes 1** and **2**).

Given that most of the girls who tested positive for a sexually transmitted disease (STD) in detention were triaged to the community in either diversion programs or nonsecure home detention, these rates of STDs and behaviors that place partners at risk constitute a significant public health challenge. Primary care providers must be aware of this issue, as it now affects youths in their practices. Clinicians will be more successful in addressing these issues if they are knowledgeable about adolescent sexuality and STD testing and treatment (see Zoon Wangu and Gale R. Burstein's article, "Adolescent Sexuality: Updates to the Sexually Transmitted Infection Guidelines," in this issue) and also comfortable and skilled in communication with adolescents about sexuality and comorbid risks (see Betsy Pfeffer and

---

Box 1
High-risk sexual behaviors

- Unprotected vaginal or anal sex
- Sex with high-risk partners (intravenous drug use, prostitution)
- Nonuse of condoms
- Multiple sexual partners
- Sex under the influence of drugs/alcohol
- Sex for money; survival sex for food/shelter

---

colleagues, "Interviewing Adolescents about Sexual Matters," in this issue). Comorbid substance use disorders in JJ-involved girls correlate with increased rates of risky sexual behavior. One study found that 96% girls with substance use disorders were sexually active; 62% had multiple partners within the preceding 3 months; and 59% had unprotected intercourse in the prior month.[40] Providers must recognize and screen for multiple interacting risks: substance use, risky sexual behaviors, home and school difficulties, and mental health issues.

SPECIAL JUVENILE JUSTICE POPULATIONS: PREGNANT/PARENTING, GANGS, SEX-TRAFFICKING, LESBIAN, GAY, BISEXUAL, TRANSGENDER
Pregnancy and Parenting in Juvenile Justice Populations

Risky sexual behavior leads to early pregnancy in the JJ population. Universal testing for pregnancy and testing for other STDs were reported by approximately 18% of the facilities surveyed in the nationwide 2004 Juvenile Justice Residential Facility (JJRF) Census. Some of the girls' residential facilities provided no pregnancy testing at all, even if the request was initiated by the girl herself. Only 4.3% of facilities tested this population for HIV. Despite the finding that 25% of these JJRFs reported housing 1 or more pregnant teen, 25% offered no obstetric services and only 85% reported that some girls received gynecologic care as necessary, based on self-reported sexual activity or suspected pregnancy.[41] The 2004 National Commission on

---

Box 2
Factors associated with risky sexual behavior

- JJ/corrections involvement
- Low self-efficacy
- Depressive self-concept
- Exposure to marital violence/physical or sexual child abuse or neglect
- School expulsion/suspension
- Difficulty communicating with partners about safe sex
- Older or more powerful partners
- Mental health comorbidity
- Substance abuse or use as self-medication
- Gang involvement

Correctional Healthcare Standards for Health Services in Juvenile Detention and Confinement Facilities, the Society for Adolescent Health and Medicine, and the American Academy of Pediatrics have all recommended STD and gynecologic care for all at-risk adolescents, especially those entering JJ facilities, which would provide unique access to this underserved population.[42–44] A survey of 1255 US JJRFs estimated a pregnancy prevalence rate of at least 2.1%, if each of the 346 facilities that reported having at least one pregnant girl in the reference month had even one pregnant girl. Obviously, this figure could be much higher. Although prenatal vitamins and options counseling should immediately be provided following a positive pregnancy test, there are limited data concerning how often this occurs. Nonjudgmental access to safe pregnancy termination services should be provided.

Given their high-risk health behaviors (substance use and smoking, high rates of mental health disorders, psychiatric medication history, STIs, HIV risk, and inadequate previous health care), these young women are at increased risk of pregnancy complications[45] and are often ill prepared to deal with parenting. Henneberger and colleagues[46] reported in 2014 that 62% of girls (71 of 114) with an incarceration history had a sub–high school level of education. Low levels of education have been linked to low occupational status, welfare dependency, and job instability.[47] At least one episode of requiring Temporary Assistance for Needy Families within 5 years following JJ involvement was reported by 21% of 700 female offenders.[48] The challenges of parenting with insufficient resources and comorbid substance use or mental health issues overwhelm many young mothers leaving JJ facilities. In one study, 62% of girls released from JJ facilities had been investigated at least once before 28 years of age by child protective services, and 42% resulted in confirmed cases of child maltreatment. Brown[49] found that nearly 50% of juvenile mothers on parole had child protection services involvement. Leve and colleagues[23] suggest that these data "underscore the potential benefit of conducting booster interventions aimed at sexual risk reduction as girls transition out of the juvenile justice system" to alter some of these negative outcomes for mothers and children.

Social Context and Influence: Impact of Gangs and Families

Social contexts surrounding the adolescent (family, school, and peers) are known to have the greatest impact on health-risk behavior.[50] Many delinquent adolescents who lack positive family influences seek surrogate family support from gang affiliation. A Department of Justice study of US JJ facilities reported that 88.5% contained gang-identified youths and that 5% to 50% of youths in JJ centers were gang involved (active members).[51,52] Gang influence promotes behaviors risky for health, augmenting already elevated rates of high-risk sexual behaviors in the JJ population. In a study of 270 detained males (aged 14–18 years; 40.7% white non-Hispanic, 39.6% African American), those who did report gang involvement in computer-assisted self-interviews were 5 to 7 times more likely to have had sexual intercourse, 3.2 times more likely to have impregnated a girl, nearly 4 times as likely to have been high on substances while having sexual intercourse, had sexual intercourse with a partner who was high, had sex with multiple partners concurrently, or did not have a condom available when wanting to have sex, compared with peers who denied gang affiliation.[53] Perceived family support, however, directly correlated with reported increased condom availability, demonstrating the positive influence of supportive families.[53]

A 2009 report by the National Council on Crime and Delinquency found that 32% of all gang members were female.[54] Gang membership confers higher sexual risk for females compared with those not in gangs: higher rates of casual sexual partnerships[53,55] and higher rates of Trichomonas and gonorrhea infections.[55] One study of

237 sexually active females aged 14 to 19 years, recruited from community venues in a Latino San Francisco neighborhood, found that Mexican-American adolescent female self-reported gang membership had no significant effect on pregnancy incidence (27.4%) over a 2-year follow-up. However, if their male partners were in a gang, that did correlate with increased pregnancy rates, even when the girls themselves were not gang affiliated.[56] A study of detained 13- to 17-year-old African American girls (N = 137), of whom 43.1% (N = 59) reported having male partners in gangs, although they themselves denied gang affiliation, identified significantly higher rates of specific high-risk sexual behaviors compared with those without gang-member partners, including decreased relationship control, higher rates of oral sex, shorter time to sex with casual sexual partners, and experiencing partner infidelity. They were also significantly less likely to have ever been tested for HIV.[57] This study recognizes the influence of both partners on sexual decision-making and advocates for sex/HIV education for both genders, using an empirically validated, partner-based intervention for African American girls and their male partners, such as HORIZONS.[58] Primary care providers should encourage inclusion of male partners in office discussions aimed at identifying and mitigating sexual risk-taking, increasing knowledge of STIs, HIV, and condom use, and improving contraceptive skills.

Because mixed-gender gangs are usually predominantly male, and the power structure within the gang advantages males and devalues females, girls are often victims of abuse: emotional, physical, and sexual. One method of gang initiation involves "sexing in", having sexual relations with multiple members of the gang. One qualitative study found that although these girls were not viewed as genuine gang members, the stigma attached to them as sexually promiscuous and weak threatened to reinforce the male gang members' view that all females are weak and exploitable. To counter this stereotype, genuine female gang members subjected "sexed-in" girls to harsh, bullying treatment. One girl sadly reported: "If you get sexed in, you have no respect. That means you gotta go ho'in' for 'em;... If you don't you gonna get your ass beat."[59]

Minor Sex Trafficking Associated with Juvenile Justice Population

History of minor sex-trafficking victimization is common among JJ-involved girls. Choi[60] found strong associations between domestic minor sex trafficking (DMST) and childhood sexual abuse, dysfunctional family environments, and interpersonal relationships that promote or normalize trading sex for money, all factors shown to be more common predictors of adolescent JJ involvement. More encounters with the JJ system were also reported as a risk for DMST in Choi's[60] review of 30 studies of DMST risk factors. A 2015 literature review of DMST found that although demographic factors (gender, race, sexual orientation, education) were not important predictors of DMST, self-identified lesbian, gay, bisexual, transgender, and queer youths, especially young men, did seem to be an at-risk group (see Joooica L. Muore and colleagues, "Sex Trafficking of Minors," in this issue).[60,61]

Nonheterosexual Youths Overrepresented in Juvenile Justice

Nonheterosexual adolescents are overrepresented in the JJ population, because they experience disproportionate criminal-justice sanctions (police stops, juvenile arrests, and convictions). This overrepresentation is not explained by rates of illegal activity or minor infractions, according to an analysis of data using the National Longitudinal Study of Adolescent Health data of adolescents in grades 7 to 12 in 1994 to 1995, subsequently followed up in 2001 to 2002.[62,63] The study found greater odds of being stopped by police (OR: 1.38; $P<.0001$) for those who report same-sex attraction and (OR: 1.53; $P<.0001$) for those who self-identify as lesbian, gay, bisexual (LGB).

School and police sanctions were more common for public display of nonheterosexual sex versus heterosexual displays. Female gender predicted higher odds of all such sanctions except school expulsion and adult arrest. Female subjects who self-identified as LGB were especially likely to experience most sanctions. Nonheterosexual youths were also more likely to receive disproportionately more severe sanctions in school, compared with heterosexual peers, including suspension and expulsion, which then increases likelihood of arrest for status offenses like truancy.[62] As a result of conflict with families over sexual orientation and verbal and physical abuse at home, 26% of nonheterosexual children become homeless runaways. Bullying in school is common. Hence, many carry weapons and engage in fights to defend themselves, putting them at risk for weapons or assault charges, even if they are the victims. They may also engage in "survival sex" (sex for money or shelter) or petty theft.

Gender Bias: Historical Discriminatory Criminalization of Female Sexuality

Some evidence exists that sexual behavior in boys and girls has historically been treated very differently by the corrections system.[64] Through the first half of the twentieth century, girls were referred to court if they were even suspected of having consensual and legal sexual intercourse. Incarceration was seen as a mandate to protect them from sexual experimentation, pregnancy, and other moral perils. Boys' sexual behavior was seen as normal experimentation. The Juvenile Justice and Delinquency Prevention Act of 1974 marked a change, requiring funded states to begin diversion and deinstitutionalization of those who committed status offences, for example, disobedience to parents or authorities, running away, truancy, or immorality. Girls, who had been historically more likely to be incarcerated for such infractions, were more impacted. Advocacy groups in the 1960s worked to redefine teenage prostitution, not as a criminal offense but as victimization and exploitation by sex trafficking. The social reform movements of the 1970s led to juvenile courts' redefinition of the "dangerous sex offender," focusing on the sexually abusive boy rather than the prostituting girl. A consensus emerged in the 1960s that perpetrators of sexual victimization, increasingly seen as a serious criminal violation, must be identified, incarcerated, and treated. Some experts assert that the system continues to disproportionately penalize girls for what are seen as unhealthy sexual behavior choices. Girls' probation often includes strict curfews at dusk, but girls trying to escape evenings of family conflict and substance abuse may run to an older boyfriend with whom the court has prohibited contact, leading to revocation of probation. The system labels her as making unhealthy choices regarding sexual relationships, rather than recognizing her action in this context as possibly the safest choice.[64]

The 2003 Prison Rape Elimination Act has led to criminalization of some behavior in juvenile detention that would be considered normative adolescent sexual experimentation and expression in the community outside. Mandated reporting to police of inappropriate touching may lead to a record as a registered sex offender, a barrier to community reentry. Once in the juvenile residential facility, normal adolescent sexual experimentation and identity explorations risk criminal penalties.[64]

SUMMARY

Acknowledging that the mission of pediatric providers is to maximize the health, welfare, and potential of all children and adolescents and recognizing that JJ-involved youths are also an integral part of our communities, medical practices, and schools, pediatric providers should seize the opportunities to mitigate risk in this hidden population (**Box 3**).

Box 3
Role for pediatric providers in care of youths with juvenile justice histories

- Screen in childhood for risk factors for justice system/court involvement
- Screen for risky sexual behaviors
- Screen for LGBT identity/bullying
- Ask about history of arrest, detention, incarceration, or probation
- Screen regularly for STIs, HIV, pregnancy, contraceptive use
- Screen for substance abuse or misuse (self-medication)
- Screen for mental illness
- Evaluate academic issues (need for IEP, ADHD treatment)
- Provide referrals for substance abuse, mental health issues
- Develop referral network to address social determinants of health: social work/agencies for example, social, financial, housing, insurance, food insecurity issues
- Obtain and share records from JJ facilities, providing continuity of care
- Use motivational interviewing to modify risk behaviors
- Use strength-based approach to interviewing

Abbreviations: ADHD, attention-deficit/hyperactivity disorder; IEP, individualized education plan; LGBT, lesbian, gay, bisexual, transgender.

REFERENCES

1. Acoca L, Stephens S, Van Vleet A. Health coverage and care for youth in the juvenile justice system: the role of medicaid and chip. Menlo Park (CA): The Kaiser Commission on Medicaid and the Uninsured; 2014.
2. Hockenberry S, Sickmund M, Saldky A. Juvenile residential facility census, 2010: selected findings. Washington, DC: OJJDP; 2013. Available at: https://www.ojjdp. gov/pubs/241134.pdf. Accessed January 12, 2017.
3. Justice Policy Institute. Building a bipartisan base for safer and smarter juvenile justice policies. 2014. Available at: http://www.justicepolicy.or/news/795. Accessed July 7, 2016.
4. Sickmund M, Sladky A, Kang W. Easy access to juvenile court statistics: 1985-2009. 2014. Available at: http://www.ojjdp.gov/oistatbb/ezajcs. Accessed July 21, 2016.
5. Snyder HN, Sickmund M. Juvenile offenders and victims: 2006 national report. Washington, DC: US Department of Justice, Office of Juvenile Justice Programs, Office of Juvenile Justice and Delinquency Prevention; 2006.
6. Holman D, Ziedenberg J. The dangers of detention: the impact of incarcerating youth in detention and other secure facilities. 2013. Available at: https://www. ncjrs.gov/App/Publications/abstract.aspx?ID=269394. Accessed July 21, 2016.
7. Barnert ES, Perry R, Morris RE. Juvenile incarceration and health. Acad Pediatr 2016;16(2):99–109.
8. Steinberg J, Grella C, Boudov M. Risky sexual behavior and negative health consequences among incarcerated female adolescents: implications for public health policy and practice. In: Sanders B, Thomas Y, Deeds BG, editors. Crime, HIV and health: intersections of criminal justice and public health concerns. New York: Springer; 2013. p. 63–79. Available at: http://dl.umsu.ac.ir/handle/ Hannan/1909. Accessed July 21, 2016.

9. Resnick M, Bearman P, Blum R, et al. Findings from the National Longitudinal Study on Adolescent Health. JAMA 1997;278(10):823–32.

10. Centers for Disease Control and Prevention (CDC). Trends in HIV-related risk behaviors among high school students–United States, 1991-2011. MMWR Morb Mortal Wkly Rep 2012;61(29):556–60.

11. Romero EG, Teplin L, McClelland G, et al. A longitudinal study of the prevalence, development, and persistence of HIV/sexually transmitted infection risk behaviors in delinquent youth: implications for health care in the community. Pediatrics 2007;119(5):e1126–41.

12. Centers for Disease Control and Prevention. Aids weekly surveillance report. Usaids program, center for infectious diseases. Atlanta (GA): Centers for disease control and Prevention; 1987.

13. CDC's HIV Surveillance Report: diagnoses of HIV infection in the United States and dependent areas, 2014. Available at: http://www.cdc.gov/hiv/pdf/library/reports/surveillance/cdc-hiv-surveillance-report-us.pdf. vol. 26. Statistics Overview | Statistics Center | HIV/AIDS | CDC www.cdc.gov/hiv/statistics/overview. Accessed July 21, 2016.

14. Wiehe SE, Rosenman MB, Aalsma MC, et al. Epidemiology of sexually transmitted infections among offenders following arrest or incarceration. Am J Public Health 2015;105(12):e26–32.

15. Aalsma MC, Ton Y, Wiehe SE, et al. The impact of delinquency on young adult sexual risk behaviors and sexually transmitted infections. J Adolesc Health 2010;46:17–24.

16. Pasko L, Chesney-Lind M. Under lock and key: trauma, marginalization, and girls' justice involvement. Justice Res Policy 2010;12(2):25–49.

17. Chesney-Lind M. Jailing "bad" girls. Fighting for girls: new perspectives on gender and violence. New York: SUNY Press;; 2010. p. 57.

18. Patino V. Getting the facts straight about girls in the juvenile justice system. Jacksonville (FL): National Council on Crime and Delinquency Center for Girls and Young Women; 2009.

19. Cauffman E, Feldman SS, Waterman J, et al. Posttraumatic stress disorder among female juvenile offenders. J Am Acad Child Adolesc Psychiatry 1998; 37:1209–16.

20. Moore E, Gaskin D, Indig D. Childhood maltreatment and post-traumatic stress disorder among incarcerated young offenders. Child Abuse Negl 2013;37:861–70.

21. Zahn MA, Agnew R, Rishbein D, et al. Causes and correlates of girls' delinquency: girls study group, understanding and responding to girls' delinquency. Washington, DC: U.S. department of Justice, Office of Justice Programs, Office of Juvenile Justice and Delinquency Prevention; 2010.

22. Leve LD, Chamberlain P. Girls in the juvenile justice system: risk factors and clinical implications. In: Pepler E, Madsen K, Webster C, et al, editors. Development and treatment of girlhood aggression. Mahwah (NJ): Erlbaum; 2005. p. 191–215.

23. Leve LD, Chamberlain P, Kim HK. Risks, outcomes and evidence-based interventions for girls in the US juvenile justice system. Clin Child Fam Psychol Rev 2015; 18:252–79.

24. Lopez V, Kopak A, Robillard M, et al. Pathways to sexual risk taking among female adolescent detainees. J Youth Adolesc 2011;40(8):945–57.

25. Goodkind S, Ng I, Sarri RC. The impact of sexual abuse in the lives of young women involved or at risk of involvement in the juvenile justice system. Violence Against Women 2006;12:456–77.

26. Wareham J, Dembo R. A longitudinal study of psychological functioning among juvenile offenders: a latent growth model analysis. Crim Justice Behav 2007;34:259–73.

27. Widom CS, Kuhns JB. Childhood victimization and subsequent risk for promiscuity, prostitution, and teenage pregnancy: a prospective study. Am J Public Health 1996;86(11):1607–12.

28. Herrera VM, McCloskey LA. Gender differences in the risk for delinquency among youth exposed to family violence. Child Abuse Negl 2001;25:1037–51.

29. Leve L, Van Ryzin M, Chamberlain P. Sexual risk behavior and STI contraction among young women with prior juvenile justice involvement. J HIV/AIDS Social Serv 2015;14(2):171–87.

30. Lederman CS, Dakof GA, Larrea MA, et al. Characteristics of adolescent females in juvenile detention. Int J Law Psychiatry 2004;27:321–37.

31. Odgers C, Robins S, Russell M. Morbidity and mortality risk among the "forgotten few": why are girls in the justice system in such poor health? Law Hum Behav 2010;34(6):429–44.

32. Kann L, Kinchen S, Shanklin SL, et al. Youth risk behavior surveillance system: United States, 2013. MMWR Morb Mortal Wkly Rep 2013;63:1–172.

33. Kann L, Lowry R, Eaton D, et al. Trends in HIV-related behaviors among high school students –United States, 1991-2011. MMWRMorbidity Mortality Weekly Rep 2012;61(29):556–60.

34. Crosby R, Salazar LF, DiClemente RJ, et al. Health risk factors among detained adolescent females. Am J Prev Med 2004;27:404–10.

35. Biswas B, Vaughn M. Really troubled girls: gender differences in risky sexual behavior and its correlates in a sample of juvenile offenders. Child Youth Serv Rev 2011;33:2386–91.

36. Dembo R, Belenko S, Childs K, et al. Drug use and sexually transmitted diseases among female and male arrested youths. J Behav Med 2009;32:129–41.

37. Kelly PJ, Blair RM, Baillargeon J, et al. Risk behaviors and the prevalence of Chlamydia in a juvenile detention facility. Clin Pediatr 2000;39:521–7.

38. Teplin LA, Mericle AA, McClelland GM, et al. HIV and AIDS risk behaviors in juvenile detainees: implications for public health policy. Am J Public Health 2003;93(6):906–12.

39. Robertson AA, Stein JA, Baird-Thomas C. Gender differences in the prediction of condom use among incarcerated juvenile offenders: testing the information-motivation-behavior skills (IMB) model. J Adolesc Health 2006;38:18–25.

40. Teplin LA, Elkington KS, McClelland GM, et al. Major mental disorders, substance use disorders, comorbidity, and HIV-AIDS risk behaviors in juvenile detainees. Psychiatr Serv 2005;56:823–8.

41. Gallagher C, Dobrin A, Douds A. A national overview of reproductive health care services for girls in juvenile justice residential facilities. Womens Health Issues 2007;17:217–26.

42. Gallagher CA, Dobrin A. Can juvenile justice detention facilities meet the call of the American Academy of Pediatrics and National Commission on Correctional Health Care? A national analysis of current practices. Pediatrics 2007;119(4):e991–1001.

43. Braverman PK, Murray PJ, American Academy of Pediatrics Committee on Adolescence. Health care for youth in the juvenile justice system. Pediatrics 2011;128(6):1219.

44. National Commission on Correctional Health Care. Standards for health services in juvenile detention and confinement facilities. Chicago: National Commission on Correctional Health Care; 2004.

45. Rizk R, Alderman E. Issues in gynecologic care for adolescent girls in the juvenile justice system. J Pediatr Adolesc Gynecol 2012;25:2–5.

46. Henneberger AK, Oudekerk BA, Reppucci ND, et al. Differential subtypes of offending among adolescent girls predict health and criminality in adulthood. Crim Justice Behav 2014;41:181–95.
47. Cauffman E. Understanding the female offender. Future Child 2008;18:119–42.
48. Bright CL, Jonson-Reid M. Young adult outcomes of juvenile court-involved girls. J Soc Serv Res 2010;36:93–106.
49. Brown M. Gender, ethnicity, and offending over the life course: women's pathways to prison in the Aloha state. Crit Criminol 2006;14:137–58.
50. Rutter M. Resilience: some conceptual considerations. J Adolesc Health 1993; 14(8):626–31.
51. Curry GD, Howell JC, Roush DW. Youth gangs in juvenile detention and corrections facilities: a national survey of juvenile detention centers (research report). Washington, DC: Office of Juvenile Justice and Delinquency Prevention; 2000.
52. Sanders B, Schneiderman JU, Loken A, et al. Gang youth as a vulnerable population for nursing intervention. Public Health Nurs 2009;26(4):346–52.
53. Voisin DR, Salazar LF, Crosby R, et al. The association between gang involvement and sexual behaviors among detained adolescent males. Sex Transm Infect 2004;80(6):440–2.
54. Glesmann C, Krisberg B, Marchionna S. Youth in gangs: who is at risk? Focus Views from the National council on Crime and Delinquency. Oakland (CA): FOCUS; 2009.
55. Wingood GM, DiClemente RJ, Crosby R, et al. Gang involvement and the health of African American female adolescents. Pediatrics 2002;110(5):e57.
56. Minnis AM, Moore JG, Doherty IA, et al. Gang exposure and pregnancy incidence among female adolescents in San Francisco: evidence for the need to integrate reproductive health with violence prevention efforts. Am J Epidemiol 2008;167(9):1102–9.
57. King KM, Voisin DR, Diclemente RJ. The relationship between male gang involvement and psychosocial risks for their female juvenile justice partners with nongang involvement histories. J Child Fam Stud 2015;24:2555. http://dx.doi.org/10.1007/s10826-014-0057-7.
58. DiClemente RJ, Wingood GM, Rose ES, et al. Efficacy of sexually transmitted disease/human immunodeficiency virus sexual risk–reduction intervention for African-American adolescent females seeking sexual health services: a randomized controlled trial. Arch Pediatr Adolesc Med 2009;163(12):1112–21.
59. Miller J. Gender and victimization risk among young women in gangs. J Res Crime Delinq 1998;35(4):429–53.
60. Choi KR. Risk factors for domestic minor sex trafficking in the United States: a literature review. J Forensic Nurs 2015;11(2):66–76.
61. Countryman-Roswurm K, Bolin BL. Domestic minor sex trafficking: assessing and reducing risk. Child Adolesc Social Work J 2014;31(6):521–38.
62. Himmelstein K, Bruckner H. Criminal-justice and school sanctions against nonheterosexual youth: a national longitudinal study. Pediatrics 2011;127(1):49–57.
63. Estrada R, Marksamer J. Lesbian, gay, bisexual and transgender young people in state custody: making the child welfare and juvenile justice systems safe for youth through litigation, advocacy and education. Temple University of the Commonwealth System of Higher Education: Temple Law Review 2006;79(2):415–38.
64. Pasko L. Damaged daughters: the history of girls' sexuality and the juvenile justice system. J Cri Law Criminol 2010;100(3):1099–130. Published by: Northwestern University School of Law Stable URL: Available at: http://www.jstor.org/stable/25766116.

Index

Note: Page numbers of article titles are in **boldface** type.

A

Abstinence
    in sexuality talks, 310
    versus LARCs, 362
Abuse, relationship. *See* Relationshiop abuse and sexual violence.
ACHES mnemonic, 348
Acne, oral contraceptives for, 352
Acyclovir, for herpes simplex virus infections, 393, 399
Adenomyosis, 336
Adolescent pregnancy, **381–388**
    adverse perinatal outcomes of, 383
    definition of, 381–382
    early diagnosis of, 382–383
    ectopic, 336
    epidemiology of, 372
    health risks of, 345
    in juvenile justice system, 455–456
    incidence of, 381–382
    office visit actions in, 383–385
    prevention of, 381–382, 386. *See also* Contraceptives.
        education on, 317
        in victims of sex trafficking, 418–419
    rates of, 360
    repeat, 385–386
    reproductive coercion for, 424–425
    risk of, 372
    unintended, emergency contraception for, **371–380**
Adolescent Reproductive and Sexual Health Education Program, 297, 299
Adolescent sexuality
    contraceptives. *See* Contraceptives.
    dating, **423–434**
    disability and, **435–449**
    dysmenorrhea, **331–342**
    human papillomavirus vaccine, **321–329**
    in juvenile justice system, **451–462**
    interviewing about, **291–304**
    parents role in information, **305–320**
    pregnancy. *See* Adolescent pregnancy.
    sex trafficking, **413–421**
    sexual violence intervention, **423–434**
    sexually transmitted infections. *See* Sexually transmitted infections.
    terminology of, 293

Pediatr Clin N Am 64 (2017) 463–474
http://dx.doi.org/10.1016/S0031-3955(17)30025-1
0031-3955/17
pediatric.theclinics.com

Moving?

Make sure your subscription moves with you!

To notify us of your new address, find your **Clinics Account Number** (located on your mailing label above your name), and contact customer service at:

Email: journalscustomerservice-usa@elsevier.com

800-654-2452 (subscribers in the U.S. & Canada)
314-447-8871 (subscribers outside of the U.S. & Canada)

Fax number: 314-447-8029

Elsevier Health Sciences Division
Subscription Customer Service
3251 Riverport Lane
Maryland Heights, MO 63043

*To ensure uninterrupted delivery of your subscription, please notify us at least 4 weeks in advance of move.

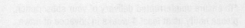

Printed and bound by CPI Group (UK) Ltd, Croydon, CR0 4YY
03/10/2024
01040495-0018